CYTOPATHOLOGY CASE REVIEW

CYTOPATHOLOGY CASE REVIEW

Christopher J. VandenBussche, MD, PhD
Assistant Professor of Pathology
The Johns Hopkins Hospital
Baltimore, Maryland

Syed Z. Ali, MD, FRCPath, FIAC
Professor of Pathology and Radiology
The Johns Hopkins Hospital
Baltimore, Maryland

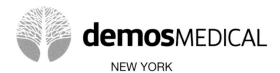

demosMEDICAL

NEW YORK

Visit our website at www.demosmedical.com

ISBN: 9781620700594
e-book ISBN: 9781617052224

Acquisitions Editor: Rich Winters
Compositor: Exeter Premedia Services Private Ltd.

Medicine is an ever-changing science. Research and clinical experience are continually expanding our knowledge, in particular our understanding of proper treatment and drug therapy. The authors, editors, and publisher have made every effort to ensure that all information in this book is in accordance with the state of knowledge at the time of production of the book. Nevertheless, the authors, editors, and publisher are not responsible for errors or omissions or for any consequences from application of the information in this book and make no warranty, expressed or implied, with respect to the contents of the publication. Every reader should examine carefully the package inserts accompanying each drug and should carefully check whether the dosage schedules mentioned therein or the contra-indications stated by the manufacturer differ from the statements made in this book. Such examination is particularly important with drugs that are either rarely used or have been newly released on the market.

Library of Congress Cataloging-in-Publication Data
VandenBussche, Christopher J., author.
Cytopathology case review / Christopher J. VandenBussche and Syed Z. Ali.
    p. ; cm.
Includes bibliographical references.
  ISBN 978-1-62070-059-4—ISBN 978-1-61705-222-4 (e-book)
 I. Ali, Syed Z., author. II. Title.
  [DNLM: 1. Cytodiagnosis—Case Reports.   2. Pathology, Clinical—Case Reports. QY 95]
  RB43
  616.07'582—dc23
                                                                                                2014038358

Special discounts on bulk quantities of Demos Medical Publishing books are available to corporations, professional associations, pharmaceutical companies, health care organizations, and other qualifying groups. For details, please contact:

Special Sales Department
Demos Medical Publishing, LLC
11 West 42nd Street, 15th Floor
New York, NY 10036
Phone: 800-532-8663 or 212-683-0072
Fax: 212-941-7842
E-mail: specialsales@demosmedical.com

Printed in the United States of America by Bradford & Bigelow.
14 15 16 17 / 5 4 3 2 1

This book is dedicated to all our past, current, and future trainees,
the major driving force behind this project.

Christopher J. VandenBussche
Syed Z. Ali

CONTENTS

FOREWORD

As the field of cytopathology becomes more complex and testing of cytologic specimens extends into the molecular realm it becomes even more important to recognize the differential diagnoses that derive from the basic morphology of the cytologic sample. *Cytopathology Case Review* allows the reader to delve into the case files of the John Hopkins University cytology department and explore the morphology and review the diagnostic possibilities. The book will be welcomed by pathology residents and fellows, cytotechnology students as well as practicing pathologists and cytotechnologists. Doctors VandenBussche and Ali share their experience and expertise in a fashion that is enjoyable and educational. The breadth of cases seen at their institution as illustrated by these cases makes the book useful for students as well as experienced cytopathologists.

The 125 cases which are presented in the following pages cover the entire gamut of cytology with representative cases from fluids, exfoliative cytology and fine needle aspirations. The cases are arranged in a random fashion in order to maximize the teaching value but may also be accessed by the sample site or type of preparation. Each case is illustrated to highlight the important cytologic features and is followed by a short pertinent history and list of potential diagnoses. On the next page is the answer with explanation and key references. These short presentations allow the reader to spend as little or as long as they wish browsing the cases and provides an easy way to review morphology or test their knowledge.

I thoroughly enjoyed sampling these cases and know that they will be of use now and well into the future.

Michael R. Henry, MD
Director of Cytopathology
Department of Laboratory Medicine
Mayo Clinic
Rochester, Minnesota

PREFACE

The field of cytopathology, while related to other fields of anatomic pathology, is rooted in its own fundamentals. While cytopathologic and histopathologic findings can often be correlated, some features found in cytologic material are absent on histology, just as histology can provide information not found in cytology. The cases presented here are intended to help focus the reader's attention on the most important cytomorphological findings.

In many instances, the images shown may suggest several possible diagnostic scenarios and the reader must choose the best answer based on limited information. This challenge is not meant to frustrate the reader, but rather to hone attention to particular findings. This format is also commonly found on standardized pathology examinations.

Regardless of whether the reader is a pathologist or cytotechnologist, a trainee may learn most from the case discussions while the more advanced reader may use the cases to test their knowledge. The readers who benefit most will be those who critically study the case images, and not necessarily the readers who answer the most questions correctly.

Several of these cases illustrated herein were modified from The Johns Hopkins Web Case Conference. We would like to acknowledge and thank Dr. Douglas P. Clark for his role as past editor of the Web Case Conference, as well as our numerous trainees that contributed cases to the conference over the years. We invite readers who enjoy these cases to participate in an updated version of the Web Case Conference, now titled "Case of the Week" and linked through our division Web page (http://pathology.jhu.edu/cytopath).

All proceedings from this book will be contributed to a cytopathology fellowship fund for education and research.

Christopher J. VandenBussche
Syed Z. Ali

CYTOPATHOLOGY CASE REVIEW

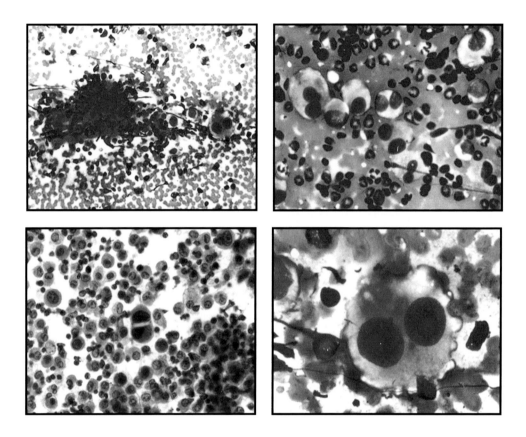

Clinical History

Pericardial fluid in a 30-year-old male with a history of a malignant neoplasm.

Choose the Best Diagnosis

    a. Metastatic adenocarcinoma

    b. Hodgkin lymphoma

    c. Reactive mesothelial cells

    d. Large cell lymphoma

    e. Melanoma

ANSWER AND BRIEF DISCUSSION

b. Hodgkin Lymphoma

This is a cellular specimen containing three populations of cells. The specimen consists predominantly of floridly reactive mesothelial cells with focal papillary formations. In addition, there are numerous small round lymphocytes in the background. The third population consists of rare, scattered, large atypical cells with abundant cytoplasm, markedly enlarged nuclei, and macronucleoli. Occasionally, these atypical cells are binucleated.

Without ancillary studies, the differential diagnosis for these large atypical cells is broad. Given the florid mesothelial proliferation, one must consider reactive mesothelial cells. However, the cells in question are distinctly larger and have a different appearance of the chromatin than the reactive mesothelial cells. A poorly differentiated adenocarcinoma could certainly present in this fashion as well and is the most common malignancy seen in an effusion sample. The clinical history is definitely helpful in this patient. This patient has a long history of Hodgkin lymphoma with multiple recurrences, most recently in the liver. The histology of the liver biopsy revealed the typical mixed lymphocytic infiltrate of Hodgkin lymphoma containing large Reed-Sternberg cells.

References

1. Das DK. Serous effusions in malignant lymphomas: a review. *Diagn Cytopathol.* 2006;34(5): 335–347.
2. McDonnell PJ, Mann RB, Bulkley BH. Involvement of the heart by malignant lymphoma: a clinicopathologic study. *Cancer.* 1982;49(5):944–951.

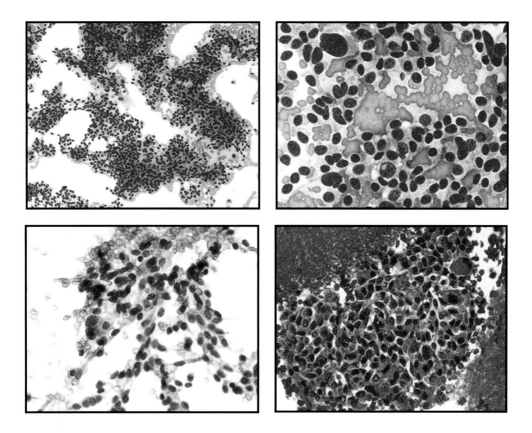

Clinical History

Fine needle aspiration of a thyroid nodule in a 51-year-old female.

Choose the Best Diagnosis

    a. Suspicious for a follicular neoplasm

    b. Medullary thyroid carcinoma

    c. Papillary thyroid carcinoma

    d. Poorly differentiated (insular) carcinoma

    e. Adenomatoid nodule

ANSWER AND BRIEF DISCUSSION

b. Medullary Thyroid Carcinoma

Cytology shows a markedly cellular smear with numerous large, loosely cohesive tissue fragments and individual cells. The nuclei of these cells are often spindled in shape, and scattered, enlarged, pleomorphic nuclei are also present. The chromatin pattern appears fine and has a neuroendocrine appearance.

The cellularity of this specimen and the lack of colloid immediately raise the suspicion of a neoplasm as opposed to an adenomatoid nodule. The presence of large sheets and enlarged nuclei suggests the possibility of papillary carcinoma; however, there is minimal overlapping of the nuclei, and nuclear chromatin is not that of papillary carcinoma. The spindled appearance of many of the nuclei is unusual for a follicular neoplasm, which typically has round nuclei and a microfollicular architecture. The combination of single cells with spindled nuclei and neuroendocrine-appearing chromatin puts medullary carcinoma at the top of the differential diagnosis. In order to confirm this diagnosis, immunohistochemical stains were performed, which revealed that the tumor was positive for calcitonin and negative for thyroglobulin, consistent with medullary thyroid carcinoma. Interestingly, the thyroid transcription factor-1 immunohistochemistry was negative. Studies have shown that the majority (>80%) of medullary carcinomas are positive for this transcription factor. If cytologic material is not available for immunohistochemical analysis, an assay to determine the patient's serum calcitonin level may be useful in establishing the diagnosis of medullary thyroid carcinoma. In young patients presenting with medullary thyroid carcinoma, a familial form of medullary thyroid carcinoma should be pursued by the clinician. Mutations in the RET oncogene may be identified in many of these familial cases.

References

1. Katoh R, Miyagi E, Nakamura N, et al. Expression of thyroid transcription factor-1 (TTF-1) in human c cells and medullary thyroid carcinomas. *Human Pathol.* 2000;31(3):386–393.
2. Hofstra RM, Landsvater RM, Ceccherini I, et al. A mutation in the RET proto-oncogene associated with multiple endocrine neoplasia type 2B and sporadic medullary thyroid carcinoma. *Nature.* 1994;367(6461):375–376.

CASE

3

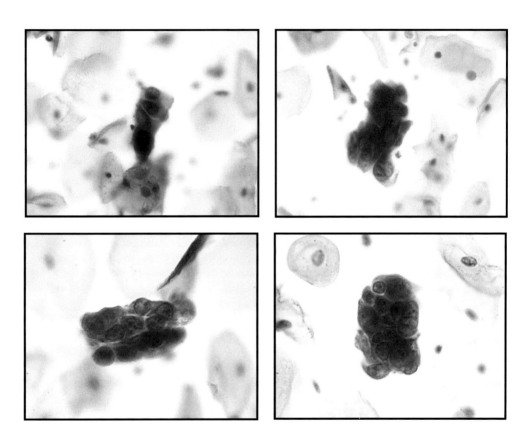

Clinical History

Liquid-based Pap test (SurePath) from a 28-year-old female.

Choose the Best Diagnosis

    a. Low-grade squamous intraepithelial lesion

    b. Negative for intraepithelial lesion or malignancy

    c. Endocervical adenocarcinoma in situ (AIS)

    d. High-grade squamous intraepithelial lesion (HSIL)

    e. Atypical squamous cells of undetermined significance (ASC-US) and atypical glandular cells (AGC)

ANSWER AND BRIEF DISCUSSION

e. ASC-US and AGC

This slide shows scattered atypical tissue fragments. These tissue fragments contain cells with enlarged nuclei arranged in a disorderly fashion within the fragment with prominent overlapping. In some fragments, the cytoplasm appears delicate and there are focal columnar, glandular features within them. Other fragments contain cells with denser cytoplasm with nuclei oriented parallel to the outline of the fragment.

Clearly, this is an abnormal Pap that should be investigated further. The question here is the possible source of the atypical cells. Are they squamous or glandular in origin? In cases such as this, atypical "glandular" cells often turn out to be a high-grade squamous dysplasia involving endocervical glands. However, in this case, there do appear to be definite glandular features such as orientation of the oval nuclei perpendicular to the outline of the fragment as well as fine delicate vacuolated cytoplasm. But other fragments have less obvious glandular features and may be squamous in origin. Because these atypical fragments lacked clear-cut glandular or squamous differentiation and because of the relative paucity of abnormal cells, this case was signed out as ASC-US and atypical glandular cells. The subsequent cervical biopsy showed an HSIL adjacent to atypical endocervical glands with enlarged overlapping nuclei, consistent with AIS.

References

1. Van Aspert-Van Erp AJM, Smedts FMM, Vooijs GP. Severe cervical glandular cell lesions with coexisting squamous cell lesions. *Cancer Cytopathol*. 2004;102(4):218–227.
2. Raab SS. Can glandular lesions be diagnosed in pap smear cytology? *Diagn Cytopathol*. 2000;23(2):127–133.

CASE

4

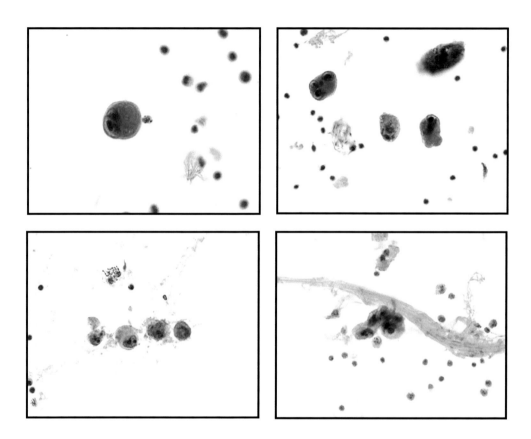

Clinical History

Pelvic fluid collection in a 56-year-old male with a history of a malignant neoplasm.

Choose the Best Diagnosis

    a. Reactive mesothelial cells

    b. Pleomorphic rhabdomyosarcoma

    c. Metastatic melanoma

    d. Anaplastic large cell lymphoma

    e. Poorly differentiated adenocarcinoma

ANSWER AND BRIEF DISCUSSION

b. Pleomorphic Rhabdomyosarcoma

This specimen contains scattered large atypical single cells. These cells contain enlarged nuclei and are sometimes multinucleated. There is abundant dense cytoplasm present. The nuclei have prominent nucleoli and markedly irregular nuclear membranes.

Based on the cytomorphology shown here, the atypical cells present are diagnostic of a malignancy. However, the exact classification of the malignancy based on cytomorphologic features is less straightforward. The lack of true tissue fragments and the presence of only single cells raise the possibility of a hematopoietic malignancy. However, the large size and abundant cytoplasm argues against this. One exception would be an anaplastic lymphoma. A poorly differentiated metastatic adenocarcinoma can present as single cells in body cavity fluids. Consequently, this diagnosis must be considered. Metastatic malignant melanoma is also in the differential diagnosis. Features suggestive of malignant melanoma include the single cell pattern, binucleation, and prominent nucleoli. Less often, sarcomas may present in body cavity effusions as single cells with large lobulated nuclei and abundant cytoplasm. In the absence of a known primary malignancy, a broad immunohistochemical panel should be applied to such a case, including antibodies against cytokeratins, HMB-45 and S100 protein, and sarcomatous elements if indicated. In this case, the patient was known to have had a pleomorphic rhabdomyosarcoma removed from the left inguinal region with positive margins 2 months prior to the pelvic fluid accumulation.

Reference

1. Abadi MA, Zakowski MF. Cytologic features of sarcomas in fluids. *Cancer*. 1998;84(2):71–76.

CASE

5

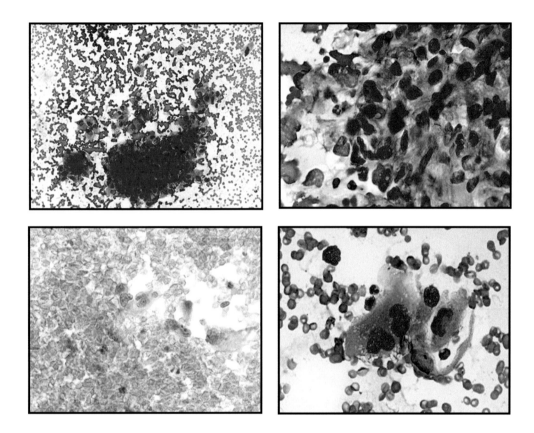

Clinical History

Fine needle aspiration (FNA) of an inguinal nodule in a 46-year-old male with a history of a malignant neoplasm.

Choose the Best Diagnosis

a. Metastatic seminoma

b. Metastatic liposarcoma

c. Clear cell sarcoma of tendon sheath

d. Metastatic urothelial carcinoma

e. Metastatic renal cell carcinoma

ANSWER AND BRIEF DISCUSSION

e. Metastatic Renal Cell Carcinoma

The smear shows scattered large cells with abundant cytoplasm that are focally vacuolated with large pleomorphic nuclei and relatively prominent nucleoli. Most of the cells appear singly or in small tissue fragments.

The microvacuoles within the cytoplasm raise the possibility that this is a "clear cell" type of tumor such as a clear cell renal cell carcinoma. However, it should also be remembered that small vacuoles may often be an artifact in some Diff-Quik-stained preparations. The delicate cytoplasm, individual nature of the cells, and pleomorphic nuclei combined with vacuoles in the cytoplasm in a soft tissue site also raise the possibility of a liposarcoma; an immunostaining panel containing cytokeratins can help distinguish these entities. In this case, the patient had a history of a clear cell renal cell carcinoma 2 years prior to this FNA. These findings were consistent with metastatic clear cell renal cell carcinoma.

Reference

1. Hughes JH, Jensen CS, Donnelly AD, et al. The role of fine-needle aspiration cytology in the evaluation of metastatic clear cell tumors. *Cancer.* 1999;87(6):380–389.

CASE

6

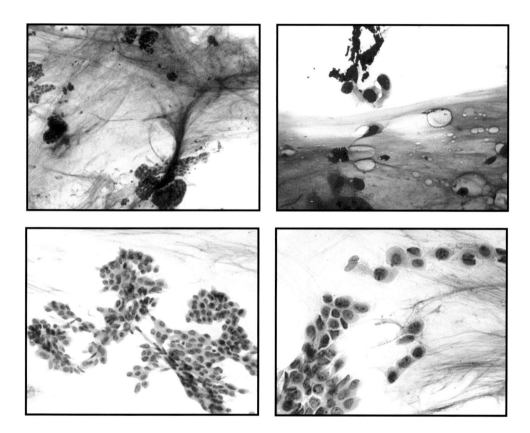

Clinical History

Fine needle aspiration (FNA) of the breast in a 53-year-old female.

Choose the Best Diagnosis

a. Intraductal papilloma

b. Fibrocystic changes

c. Fibroadenoma with mucinous change

d. Ductal carcinoma with mucinous features

e. Mucocele

ANSWER AND BRIEF DISCUSSION

d. Ductal Carcinoma With Mucinous Features

These smears contain abundant mucin in the background. Scattered amid the mucin are large cells arranged predominantly in tissue fragments, with occasional single cells present as well. The cells have relatively large nuclei with prominent nucleoli.

The presence of abundant mucin in a breast FNA certainly raises the concern of a mucinous carcinoma, such as a colloid carcinoma. Other things to be considered include a mucocele of the breast or a fibroadenoma with mucinous change. In this case, the nuclear size and presence of occasional single atypical cells puts the diagnosis of colloid carcinoma at the top of the differential diagnosis. The characteristic myoepithelial cells and typical ductal fragments seen in a fibroadenoma are not present here, and the amount of mucin is beyond that expected with a focal mucinous change within a fibroadenoma. Mucoceles should only contain muciphages and rare-to-no ductal epithelium.

References

1. Duane GB, Kanter MH, Branigan T, Chang C. A morphologic and morphometric study of cells from colloid carcinoma of the breast obtained by fine needle aspiration. Distinction from other breast lesions. *Acta Cytol*. 1987;31:742–750.
2. Masood S, Loya A, Khalbuss W. Is core needle biopsy superior to fine-needle aspiration biopsy in the diagnosis of papillary breast lesions? *Diagn Cytopathol*. 2003;28(6):329–334.

CASE

7

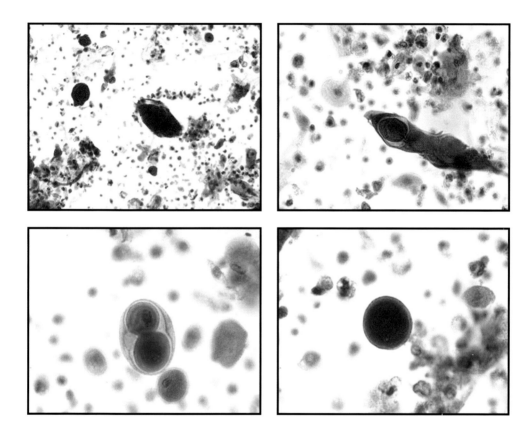

Clinical History

Voided urine specimen in a 78-year-old female with flank pain.

Choose the Best Diagnosis

    a. Carcinoma with extensive squamous differentiation

    b. Squamous metaplasia with associated schistosomiasis

    c. Changes associated with urolithiasis

    d. Human papillomavirus-induced cellular changes

    e. Granulomatous cystitis and atypical squamous cells

ANSWER AND BRIEF DISCUSSION

a. Carcinoma With Extensive Squamous Differentiation

Cytology shows the presence of numerous atypical keratinized cells. These cells are large, brightly orangeophilic, and contain large irregular hyperchromatic nuclei. There is abundant keratinaceous debris in the background as well. Focally, there are cells that appear to have enlarged abnormal nuclei with a much higher N/C ratio without obvious keratinization to the cytoplasm.

The presence of keratinized squamous cells within a urine specimen raises the possibility of squamous metaplasia within the bladder, which can be associated with schistosomiasis. However, this patient is not from an endemic area. Although the abundance of material in this case argues for an origin within the urinary tract, a gynecologic primary should also be considered. This abnormal voided urine cytology prompted a clinical workup, which revealed that the bladder was normal. However, the renal pelvis was markedly abnormal. A nephrectomy was performed that revealed a high-grade papillary urothelial carcinoma within the renal pelvis with foci of squamous differentiation. There is no known history of lithiasis in this patient.

References

1. Guo CC, Fine SW, Epstein JI. Noninvasive squamous lesions in the urinary bladder: a clinicopathologic analysis of 29 cases. *Am J Surg Pathol*. 2006;30(7):883–891.
2. Hattori M, Nishimura Y, Toyonaga M, Kakinuma H, Matsumoto K, Ohbu M. Cytological significance of abnormal squamous cells in urinary cytology. *Diagn Cytopathol*. 2012;40(9): 798–803.
3. Owens CL, Ali SZ. Atypical squamous cells in exfoliative urinary cytology: clinicopathologic correlates. *Diagn Cytopathol*. 2005;33(6):394–398.

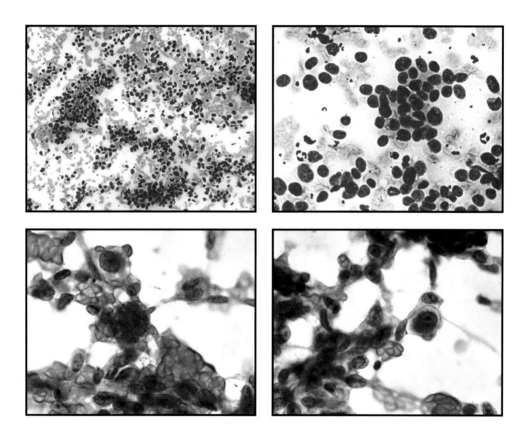

Clinical History

Lung fine needle aspiration in a 78-year-old female with a history of a salivary gland tumor 30 years ago and surgery for hemorrhoids 1 year ago.

Choose the Best Diagnosis

a. Metastatic leiomyosarcoma

b. Metastatic malignant melanoma

c. Metastatic myoepithelioma

d. Small cell carcinoma of the lung

e. Non-Hodgkin lymphoma

ANSWER AND BRIEF DISCUSSION

b. Metastatic Malignant Melanoma

Cytology shows loosely cohesive fragments containing cells with prominent spindled morphology. Focally, there is some pleomorphism among the nuclei. Careful examination reveals focal intracytoplasmic pigment deposition within the cells.

This lesion falls into the general category of a spindle cell neoplasm. Of course, this raises the possibility of a sarcoma, possibly a leiomyosarcoma, either primary in the lung or a metastatic lesion. Although the chromatin is not entirely consistent with a neuroendocrine neoplasm, this should probably also be considered in the differential diagnosis (peripheral carcinoid). As it turns out, the reported "hemorrhoid" surgery was actually for malignant melanoma of the skin adjacent to the anus. Given this history and the presence of multiple lesions in the lung, this is consistent with metastatic malignant melanoma.

References

1. Slagel DD, Powers CN, Melaragno MJ, Geisinger KR, Frable WJ, Silverman JF. Spindle-cell lesions of the mediastinum: diagnosis by fine-needle aspiration biopsy. *Diagn Cytopathol.* 1997;17(3): 167–176.
2. Hummel P, Cangiarella JF, Cohen JM, Yang G, Waisman J, Chhieng DC. Transthoracic fine-needle aspiration biopsy of pulmonary spindle cell and mesenchymal lesions: a study of 61 cases. *Cancer.* 2001;93(3):187–198.

CASE

9

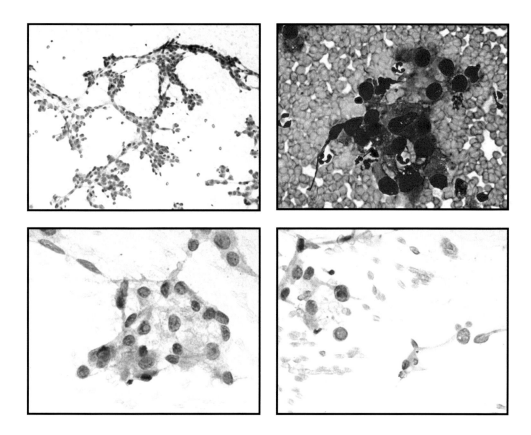

Clinical History

Fine needle aspiration of a liver lesion in a 43-year-old black male.

Choose the Best Diagnosis

    a. Metastatic adenocarcinoma, consistent with colonic primary

    b. Metastatic malignant melanoma

    c. High-grade neuroendocrine carcinoma

    d. Intrahepatic cholangiocarcinoma

    e. Poorly differentiated hepatocellular carcinoma (HCC)

ANSWER AND BRIEF DISCUSSION

e. Poorly Differentiated Hepatocellular Carcinoma (HCC)

This is a very cellular specimen containing both tissue fragments and individual naked nuclei. The naked nuclei are large and round with prominent nucleoli and focal striking vacuolation. The tissue fragments are composed of similar cells with a moderate amount of cytoplasm.

This is clearly a poorly differentiated malignant neoplasm due to the nuclear size and pleomorphism. In these cases, the question often arises as to whether the neoplasm is a primary HCC or a metastatic poorly differentiated carcinoma. The presence of numerous round naked nuclei favors an HCC. In addition, the striking vacuolation present in the nuclei is felt to be consistent with a hepatitis B-associated HCC. The serum alpha-fetoprotein level in this patient was greater than 26,000, consistent with an HCC.

Reference

1. Takenaka A, Kaji I, Kasugai H, et al. Usefulness of diagnostic criteria for aspiration cytology of hepatocellular carcinoma. *Acta Cytol.* 1999;43(4):610–616.

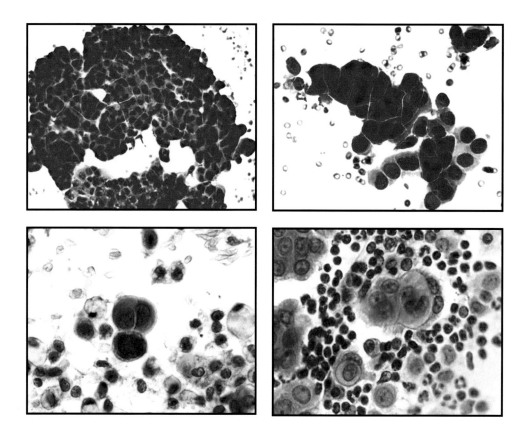

Clinical History

Fine needle aspiration of a pleural-based mass in the right lung of a 65-year-old male with a history of left lung adenocarcinoma and prostatic cancer.

Choose the Best Diagnosis

a. Squamous cell carcinoma

b. Adenocarcinoma of the lung

c. Malignant mesothelioma

d. Metastatic prostatic adenocarcinoma

e. Reactive mesothelial cells

ANSWER AND BRIEF DISCUSSION

c. Malignant Mesothelioma

Cytology shows the presence of numerous tissue fragments containing markedly atypical epithelioid cells. These cells have enlarged nuclei with high (N/C) ratios. The nuclei do not contain prominent nucleoli. There is no obvious squamous differentiation; however, there are focal areas suggesting glandular features.

This is obviously a malignant process; however, the origin of the tumor is open for discussion. The differential diagnosis includes a second lung carcinoma, probably an adenocarcinoma, developing in the contralateral lung (or a metastasis from the previous lung adenocarcinoma). Given the patient's history, a metastatic prostatic carcinoma is also in the differential. Although it seems clinically less likely, a third primary should also be considered, given the pleural-based location of this lesion. A series of immunohistochemical stains were performed on the specimen to narrow down the differential diagnosis. First, cytokeratin 7 and 20 were analyzed. One would anticipate that cytokeratin 7 would be positive and cytokeratin 20 would be negative for both lung and epithelioid mesothelioma. Prostate carcinoma should be negative for both of these cytokeratins. Prostate-specific antigen and NKX3.1 can help identify metastatic prostatic carcinoma. A panel of immunostains were also performed to distinguish between a lung adenocarcinoma and a mesothelioma. These stains included LeuM1 (CD15), mCEA, p53, and thyroid transcription factor-1 (TTF-1). One would anticipate LeuM1 and mCEA to be negative in mesotheliomas, which was the case in this tumor. The TTF-1 immunostaining in this case was negative, consistent with mesothelioma. A p53 stain was also performed, which showed abundant positive nuclear staining. At least 40% of mesotheliomas show immunostaining for p53, which reflects a mutation in the p53 gene causing persistence and accumulation of the mutant form of p53 within the nucleus. Of course, a significant percentage of lung adenocarcinomas also have p53 mutations, so immunostaining for this protein does not distinguish between these two entities. A calretinin stain was focally positive.

Reference

1. Whitaker D. The cytology of malignant mesothelioma. *Cytopathology*. 2000;11(3):139–151.

CASE

11

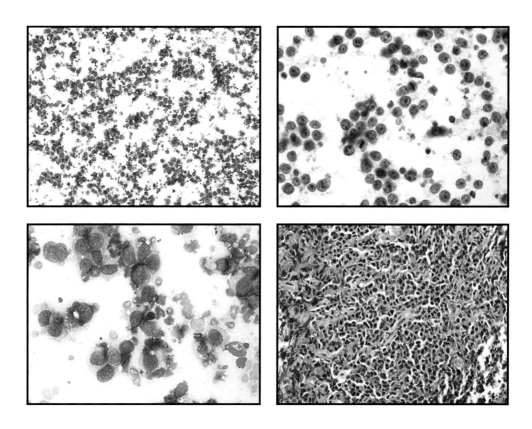

Clinical History

Fine needle aspiration of a destructive lesion of the left hip in an HIV+ 46-year-old male.

Choose the Best Diagnosis

    a. Metastatic malignant melanoma

    b. Large cell lymphoma

    c. Metastatic poorly differentiated adenocarcinoma

    d. Findings consistent with avascular necrosis

    e. Mycobacterium tuberculosis involving bone (Pott's disease)

ANSWER AND BRIEF DISCUSSION

b. Large Cell Lymphoma

This is a cellular specimen containing predominantly individual cells. These cells appear as naked nuclei or with scant cytoplasm. The nuclei are enlarged, but generally round, and have large central prominent nucleoli. There is necrosis and apoptotic debris in the background.

The differential diagnosis for solitary bony lesions in HIV+ individuals is broad and includes both neoplastic and infectious etiologies. In this case, the presence of a monotonous population of large, atypical cells favors a neoplastic process. Flow cytometric immunophenotyping was noncontributory due to a large amount of necrotic debris. Due to a prominent single-cell pattern and presence of prominent nucleoli, a metastatic malignant melanoma was also considered; however, the morphologic appearance is not entirely typical, and immunohistochemical stain for HMB-45 was negative. We have identified several HIV+ patients who have presented with widely metastatic poorly differentiated lung adenocarcinoma. Therefore, this is also in the differential diagnosis. However, the morphologic appearance is not entirely consistent with this diagnosis, and stains for cytokeratins including AE1/AE3, CAM 5.2, and EMA were all negative. Immunohistochemical stains did, however, support the initial impression of malignant lymphoma, showing positive staining for CLA and CD20.

References

1. Verstovsek G, Chakraborty S, Ramzy I, Jorgensen JL. Large b-cell lymphomas: fine-needle aspiration plays an important role in initial diagnosis of cases which are falsely negative by flow cytometry. *Diagn Cytopathol*. 2002;27(5):282–285.
2. Bommer KK, Ramzy I, Mody D. Fine-needle aspiration biopsy in the diagnosis and management of bone lesions: a study of 450 cases. *Cancer*. 1997;81(3):148–156.

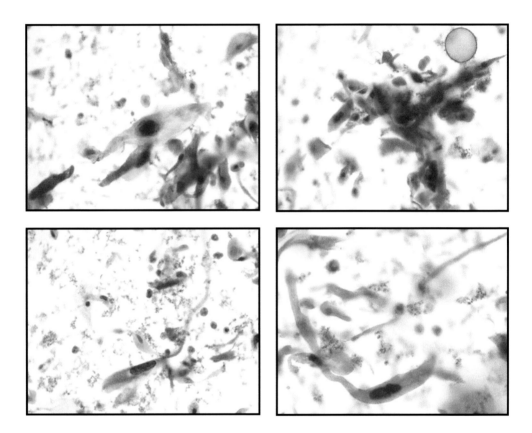

Clinical History

This is a liquid-based Pap test (SurePath) done on an ecto/endocervical sample from a 52-year-old black female.

Choose the Best Diagnosis

    a. Squamous cell carcinoma of the cervix

    b. High-grade squamous intraepithelial lesion

    c. Atypical squamous cells of undetermined significance, with extensive atypical parakeratosis

    d. Atypical glandular cells

    e. Negative for intraepithelial lesion or malignancy

ANSWER AND BRIEF DISCUSSION

a. Squamous Cell Carcinoma of the Cervix

At low power, this monolayer preparation contains abundant keratinized cells that are spindled in shape. The background contains extensive altered blood. On higher power, many of these spindled keratinized cells are anucleated. The nucleated cells are markedly atypical, with striking hyperchromasia of the nuclei along with some nuclear enlargement and angulation of the nuclear outlines. In addition to the altered blood in the background, there are several tissue fragments present that suggest necrosis.

Even at the low power, this is a very concerning specimen because of the abundant altered blood in the background, suggestive of a tumor diathesis. The markedly atypical keratinizing cells are highly suspicious for squamous carcinoma. The necrosis and altered blood raise the possibility of invasion.

Reference

1. Sherman ME, Dasgupta A, Schiffman M, Nayar R, Solomon D. The Bethesda Interobserver Reproducibility Study (BIRST): a web-based assessment of the Bethesda 2001 System for classifying cervical cytology. *Cancer*. 2007;111(1):15–25.

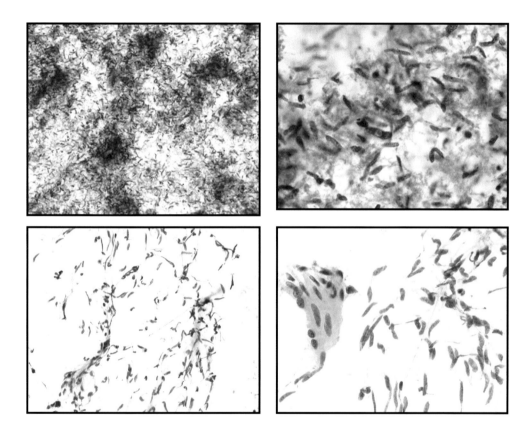

Clinical History

Fine needle aspiration of a submucosal gastric mass in a 73-year-old black male.

Choose the Best Diagnosis

    a. Pseudosarcoma

    b. Gastrointestinal stromal tumor (GIST)

    c. Schwannoma

    d. Spindle cell neoplasm, favor leiomyosarcoma

    e. Spindle cell neoplasm, favor solitary fibrous tumor

ANSWER AND BRIEF DISCUSSION

b. Gastrointestinal Stromal Tumor (GIST)

This is an extremely cellular specimen containing numerous individual cells with markedly elongated nuclei. Nuclear pleomorphism is minimal, with only occasional large nuclei present. Cells have barely intact scant cytoplasm. Also present is somewhat fibrillar-appearing background material.

This specimen has the general appearance of a spindle cell neoplasm. The most common spindle cell neoplasm of the stomach is the GIST. Other rare neoplasms such as a schwannoma may also be considered. GISTs represent a heterogeneous group of mesenchymal tumors whose behavior varies from benign to malignant. While originally thought to be of true smooth muscle origin, molecular markers suggested they may originate from the interstitial cells of Cajal, which have both myoid and neural features. These tumors can be divided into spindle cell and epithelioid types. Immunohistochemistry can be helpful in making the diagnosis of GIST. Typically, these tumors are positive for BCL2 and often CD34. In addition, this neoplasm expresses the c-KIT (CD117) molecule. This molecule is a growth factor receptor with tyrosine kinase activity that may play a role in the tumorigenesis of this neoplasm. Gain-of-function mutations have been identified in this gene and may be associated with more malignant behavior.

Reference

1. Li SQ, O'Leary TJ, Buchner SB, et al. Fine needle aspiration of gastrointestinal stromal tumors. *Acta Cytol*. 2001;45(1):9–17.

CASE

14

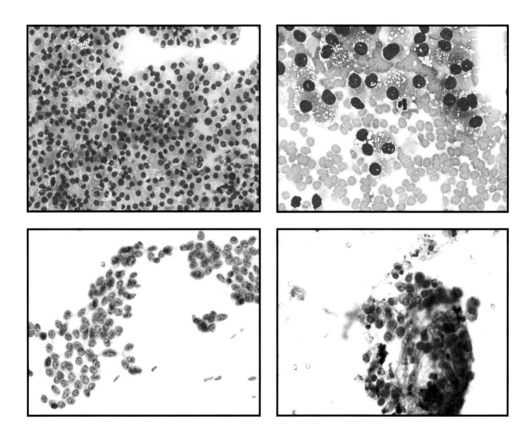

Clinical History

Fine needle aspiration of a pancreatic mass in a 78-year-old male.

Choose the Best Diagnosis

a. Well-differentiated pancreatic neuroendocrine tumor (PanNET)

b. Pancreatic ductal adenocarcinoma

c. Malignant lymphoma

d. Normal pancreatic acinar tissue

e. Plasmacytoma

ANSWER AND BRIEF DISCUSSION

a. Well-Differentiated Pancreatic Neuroendocrine Tumor (PanNET)

The smears are hypercellular and contain scattered single cells and small irregular tissue fragments containing relatively small cells with high N/C ratios. The nuclei are monotonous and oval, and on the Papanicolaou stain, have a characteristic neuroendocrine-type chromatin. Immunohistochemical stains for neuroendocrine markers were attempted, but displayed a high background and were noncontributory in this case.

The smear contains cells that are significantly smaller than the typical ductal adenocarcinoma or acinar cell carcinoma of the pancreas. The neoplastic cells have a characteristic eccentric nuclear placement (plasmacytoid morphology). Numerous fine lipid vacuoles are also observed in the cytoplasm, another feature often observed in PanNETs.

Reference

1. Chatzipantelis P, Salla C, Konstantinou P, Karoumpalis I, Sakellariou S, Doumani I. Endoscopic ultrasound-guided fine-needle aspiration cytology of pancreatic neuroendocrine tumors: a study of 48 cases. *Cancer.* 2008;114(4):255–262.

CASE

15

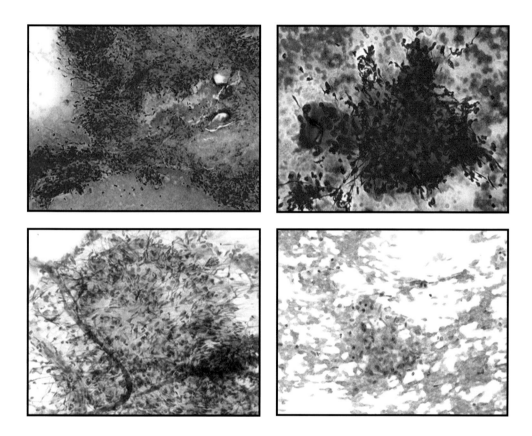

Clinical History

Fine needle aspiration of an ulcerated, draining neck lesion in a 57-year-old female.

Choose the Best Diagnosis

a. Sarcoidosis

b. Ulcerating tuberculous infection (scrofula)

c. Synovial sarcoma

d. Mucoepidermoid carcinoma

e. Squamous cell carcinoma, necrotic

ANSWER AND BRIEF DISCUSSION

b. Ulcerating Tuberculous Infection (Scrofula)

This specimen contains numerous multinucleated giant cells (Langhans type) as well as intermixed lymphocytes and aggregates of epithelioid histiocytes and lymphocytes, consistent with granulomata. No malignancy is identified.

This case clearly shows granulomatous inflammation. The etiology of the granulomatous inflammation is not apparent based on the cytomorphology alone and includes mycobacterial and fungal infections. In this case, an acid-fast stain on one smear revealed numerous acid-fast bacilli. Speciation of these mycobacteria is not possible on morphology alone, so cultures were obtained. Interestingly, microbial cultures were negative, demonstrating the importance of careful cytologic examination. This case is clinically consistent with scrofula, an ulcerating tuberculous infection of the cervical lymph nodes.

References

1. Ellison E, Lapuerta P, Martin SE. Fine needle aspiration diagnosis of mycobacterial lymphadenitis. Sensitivity and predictive value in the United States. *Acta Cytol*. 1999;43(2):153–157.
2. Fontanilla JM, Barnes A, von Reyn CF. Current diagnosis and management of peripheral tuberculous lymphadenitis. *Clin Infect Dis*. 2011;53(6):555–562.

CASE

16

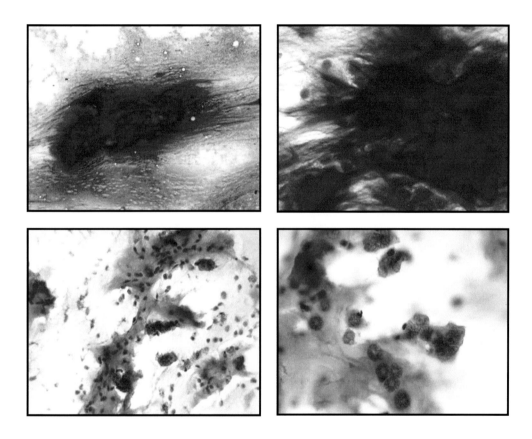

Clinical History

Fine needle aspiration of a right parotid mass in a 47-year-old male.

Choose the Best Diagnosis

    a. Chronic sialadenitis

    b. Adenoid cystic carcinoma

    c. Pleomorphic adenoma

    d. Basal cell adenoma

    e. Warthin tumor

ANSWER AND BRIEF DISCUSSION

c. Pleomorphic Adenoma

These smears contain abundant fibrillary metachromatic-staining acellular matrix material along with scattered myoepithelial type cells in the background. There is also abundant crystalline material in the background.

These findings are classic for pleomorphic adenoma. This crystalline debris is most obvious on the Papanicolaou-stained material and has a striking radial configuration and in areas a petal-shaped morphology consistent with the so-called tyrosine-rich crystalloid. The etiology and significance of these crystalloids are not known. Some investigators have also found calcium, phosphorus, and magnesium within these crystalloids. Other crystalline structures have been described in pleomorphic adenomas, but have more of a polyhedral, multifaceted appearance.

References

1. Nasuti JF, Gupta PK, Fleisher SR, LiVolsi VA. Nontyrosine crystalloids in salivary gland lesions: report of seven cases with fine-needle aspiration cytology and follow-up surgical pathology. *Diagn Cytopathol.* 2000;22(3):167–171.
2. Humphrey PA, Ingram P, Tucker A, Shelburne JD. Crystalloids in salivary gland pleomorphic adenomas. *Arch of Pathol Lab Med.* 1989;113(4):390–393.

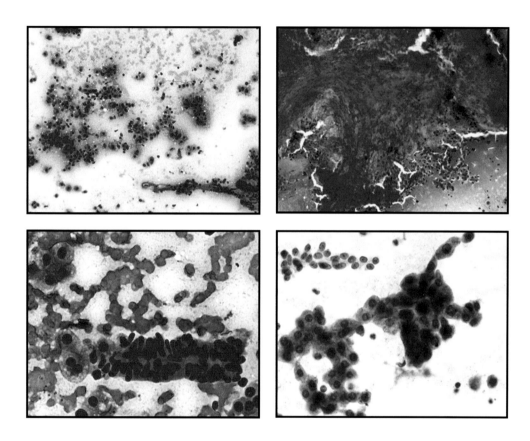

Clinical History

Ultrasound-guided liver fine needle aspiration (FNA) in a 41-year-old female.

Choose the Best Diagnosis

a. Metastatic breast carcinoma

b. Hepatocellular carcinoma (HCC)

c. Hepatic adenoma

d. Consistent with focal nodular hyperplasia

e. Normal hepatic tissue

ANSWER AND BRIEF DISCUSSION

d. Consistent With Focal Nodular Hyperplasia

The interpretation of focal nodular hyperplasia is often extremely difficult on limited FNA samples and is usually considered "a diagnosis of exclusion" after careful analysis of clinical, radiological, and serum alpha-fetoprotein (AFP) findings.

These smears reveal numerous benign-appearing hepatocytes, fragments of fibrous tissue, and scattered benign biliary epithelial cells.

At first glance, this is the cytology of a normal liver. The hepatocytes are relatively small with small nuclei and abundant cytoplasm. There are no scattered atypical naked nuclei present, which is a feature of HCC. The architecture of the existing fragments does not look atypical in that there do not appear to be large atypical sheets of hepatocytes without intervening sinusoids and ducts. So, while a well-differentiated HCC can sometimes be difficult to exclude, there do not appear to be overt features in this specimen. Often, the differential diagnosis of a solitary nodule in a relatively young woman is that of a hepatic adenoma versus focal nodular hyperplasia. The key distinguishing features in focal nodular hyperplasia include normal bile duct epithelium and fibrous tissue. The latter represents the dense central fibrous scar of focal nodular hyperplasia. In this patient, the presence of both features favors a diagnosis of focal nodular hyperplasia. Of course, in such cases where atypia is minimal, serum markers for AFP may also be useful in ruling out a well-differentiated HCC. It is possible that the radiologist simply missed the lesion, so a diagnosis of hepatic adenoma or focal nodular hyperplasia must be rendered very carefully on a cytologic specimen and is typically worded as "consistent with focal nodular hyperplasia, recommend careful radiographic correlation to ensure adequate sampling."

References

1. Wee A. Fine needle aspiration biopsy of the liver. Algorithmic approach and current issues in the diagnosis of hepatocellular carcinoma. *CytoJournal.* 2005;2:7.
2. Ruschenburg I, Droese M. Fine needle aspiration cytology of focal nodular hyperplasia of the liver. *Acta Cytol.* 1989;33(6):857–860.

CASE

18

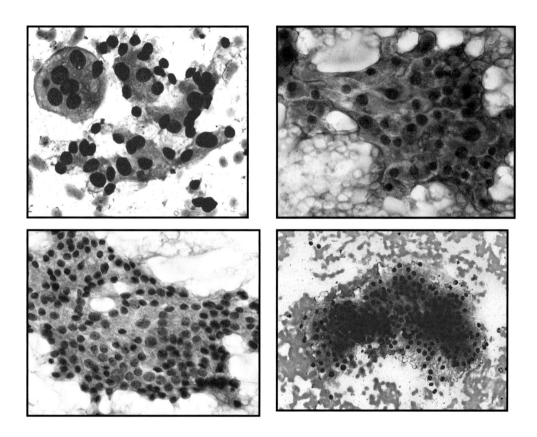

Clinical History

Ultrasound-guided fine needle aspiration of a thyroid nodule in a 72-year-old female.

Choose the Best Diagnosis

    a. Papillary thyroid carcinoma, oncocytic variant

    b. Suspicious for a follicular neoplasm, Hurthle cell type

    c. Consistent with Graves' disease

    d. Adenomatoid nodule

    e. Medullary thyroid carcinoma

CASE 18 ■ 35

ANSWER AND BRIEF DISCUSSION

c. Consistent With Graves' Disease

These slides are moderately cellular and contain follicular cells with abundant granular cytoplasm. The follicular cells are notable for focal nuclear enlargement and pleomorphism. No intranuclear grooves or inclusions are identified.

At first glance, this case appears to represent a typical adenomatoid nodule. However, closer examination reveals that there is random nuclear enlargement within several of the follicular clusters. Such nuclear enlargements raise the possibility of a neoplastic process such as papillary carcinoma. However, other nuclear features are not consistent with that of papillary carcinoma. There are no nuclear grooves or inclusions identified and the chromatin is coarser than the typical papillary carcinoma, plus this nuclear enlargement appears somewhat random in nature. Fortunately, we were given clinical information that provided two possible explanations for this nuclear atypia. First, this patient suffered from Graves' disease, which can alone produce some nuclear enlargement. In addition, this patient had been treated with radioactive iodine for her Graves' disease. Radioactive iodine therapy is known to induce such random atypia within the follicular epithelium. It is important for the cytopathologist to be aware of this clinical information and to not overreact to nuclear enlargement in this setting.

References

1. Jayaram G, Singh B, Marwaha RK. Grave's disease. Appearance in cytologic smears from fine needle aspirates of the thyroid gland. *Acta Cytol.* 1989;33(1):36–40.
2. Baloch ZW, Cibas ES, Clark DP, et al. The National Cancer Institute thyroid fine needle aspiration state of the science conference: a summation. *CytoJournal.* 2008;5:6.

CASE

19

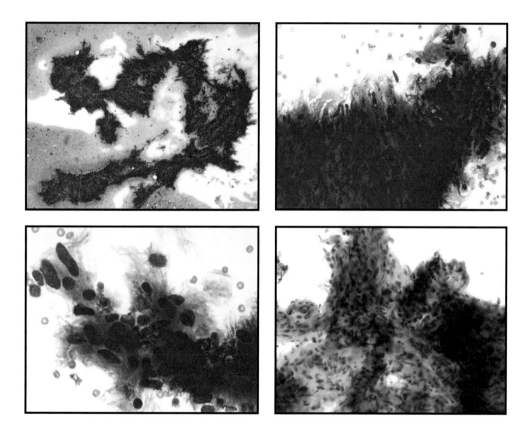

Clinical History

Fine needle aspiration in a 41-year-old male with a 1-cm nodule anterior to the lateral mandible.

Choose the Best Diagnosis

a. Benign fibrous histiocytoma

b. Leiomyoma

c. Traumatic neuroma

d. Schwannoma

e. Malignant peripheral nerve sheath tumor

ANSWER AND BRIEF DISCUSSION

d. Schwannoma

This is a moderately cellular specimen composed predominantly of large irregular tissue fragments. Within these fragments are cells with spindle-shaped nuclei and interposed acellular matrix. There are occasional naked spindled nuclei in the background.

This represents a spindle cell neoplasm. It is relatively cohesive and has minimal pleomorphism. The nuclei have focal pointed ends and a wavy character suggestive of neural origin. In addition, the acellular material in between the nuclei has a very fibrillar appearance. The differential diagnosis in this unusual anatomic site is somewhat broad and includes fibrous lesions such as a neurofibroma or a benign fibrous histiocytoma as well as a traumatic neuroma. On the cell block material (not shown here), there was an area that appears to represent a Verocay body with the Antoni A (cellular) and Antoni B (less cellular) areas, typical of a schwannoma.

References

1. Chi AC, Carey J, Muller S. Intraosseous schwannoma of the mandible: a case report and review of the literature. *Oral surgery, oral medicine, oral pathology, oral radiology, and endodontics.* 2003;96(1):54–65.
2. Yu GH, Sack MJ, Baloch Z, Gupta PK. Difficulties in the fine needle aspiration (FNA) diagnosis of schwannoma. *Cytopathology.* 1999;10(3):186–194.

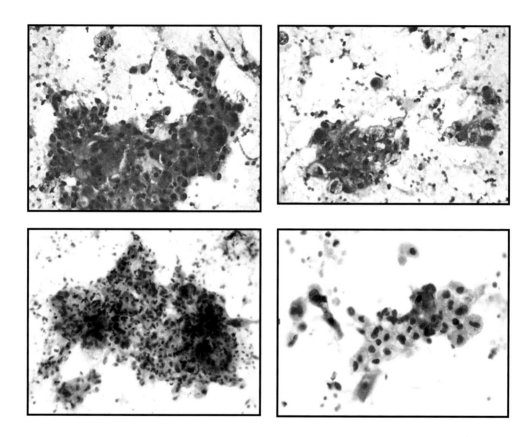

Clinical History

Parotid fine needle aspiration (FNA) in an 85-year-old male with a remote history of a moderately differentiated adenocarcinoma of the rectum as well as a remote history of an adenocarcinoma of the prostate, Gleason score 3 + 3 = 6.

Choose the Best Diagnosis

a. Metastatic squamous cell carcinoma

b. Squamous cell carcinoma of the parotid

c. Warthin tumor with squamous metaplasia

d. Mucoepidermoid carcinoma (MEC), high grade

e. Epidermal inclusion cyst with reactive atypia

ANSWER AND BRIEF DISCUSSION

d. Mucoepidermoid Carcinoma (MEC), High Grade

The FNA specimen reveals a moderately cellular specimen containing markedly atypical epithelial fragments with large nuclei and prominent nucleoli. There are numerous vacuolated cells in the background focally in association with the atypical epithelium.

While one might initially consider the possibility that this is a cystic lesion lined by reactive squamous epithelium, the atypia within the epithelium and the abundance of it favor a high-grade epithelial malignancy. In areas there is obvious squamous differentiation in the epithelial fragments. Given the patient's history of prostatic and rectal adenocarcinomas, a metastatic lesion should be considered initially. While treated prostate carcinoma can undergo squamous metaplasia in metastatic lesions, this clinical picture would be very unusual. There is no mention of squamous differentiation within the patient's previous rectal carcinoma, so a metastasis from one of these sites seems unlikely. A primary squamous carcinoma of the salivary gland is rare, but should be considered in the differential diagnosis along with a metastatic squamous carcinoma from another site such as the oropharynx or lung. However, the presence of vacuolated cells in the background and particularly vacuolated cells in intimate association with the epithelial fragments raises the possibility of a high-grade MEC of the parotid.

References

1. Al-Khafaji BM, Nestok BR, Katz RL. Fine-needle aspiration of 154 parotid masses with histologic correlation: ten-year experience at the University of Texas MD Anderson Cancer Center. *Cancer*. 1998;84(3):153–159.
2. Stewart CJ, MacKenzie K, McGarry GW, Mowat A. Fine-needle aspiration cytology of salivary gland: a review of 341 cases. *Diagn Cytopathol*. 2000;22(3):139–146.

CASE

21

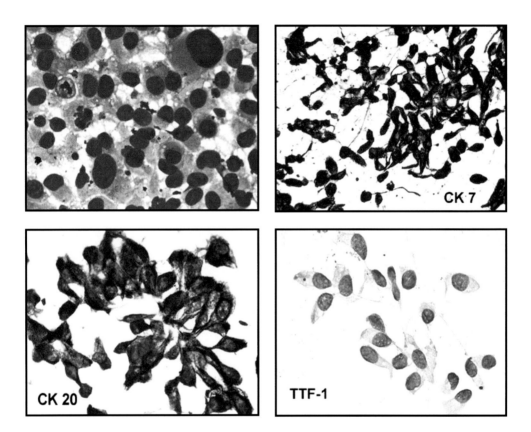

Clinical History

Fine needle aspiration of a lung nodule, pleural-based, in a 70-year-old female with a remote history of colonic adenocarcinoma and a more recent history of high-grade invasive urothelial carcinoma.

Choose the Best Diagnosis

 a. Metastatic colonic adenocarcinoma

 b. Metastatic urothelial carcinoma

 c. Adenocarcinoma of the lung

 d. Malignant mesothelioma

 e. Reactive changes

ANSWER AND BRIEF DISCUSSION

b. Metastatic Urothelial Carcinoma

This is a markedly cellular and relatively monotonous sample. The cells are quite discohesive, contain a moderate amount of cytoplasm, and have a somewhat enlarged, eccentrically placed nucleus.

This is clearly a non-small cell carcinoma, but the distinction among a primary lung adenocarcinoma, an epithelioid mesothelioma (given the pleural-based nature), a metastatic poorly differentiated colonic carcinoma, and a metastatic poorly differentiated urothelial carcinoma is somewhat challenging based on the cytomorphology. Given the morphology alone, the discohesive nature and the relatively round nuclei (as opposed to columnar shaped cells and oval nuclei) argue against a metastatic colonic adenocarcinoma. Immunohistochemical studies can be employed to distinguish among the remaining entities. In this case, the tumor cells are positive for cytokeratin 7 and 20 and negative for calretinin and thyroid transcription factor-1 (TTF-1). A primary lung adenocarcinoma would tend to be cytokeratin 7 positive and cytokeratin 20 negative, and positive for TTF-1. GATA-3 is often positive in urothelial carcinomas, but would be negative in adenocarcinoma of the lung and colon. A mesothelioma would likely express calretinin.

References

1. Siddiqui MT, Seydafkan S, Cohen C. GATA3 expression in metastatic urothelial carcinoma in fine needle aspiration cell blocks. *Diagn Cytopathol.* 2014;42(9):809–815. doi:10.1002/dc.23131.
2. Gruver AM, Amin MB, Luthringer DJ. Selective immunohistochemical markers to distinguish between metastatic high-grade urothelial carcinoma and primary poorly differentiated invasive squamous cell carcinoma of the lung. *Arch Pathol Lab Med.* 2012;136(11):1339–1346.

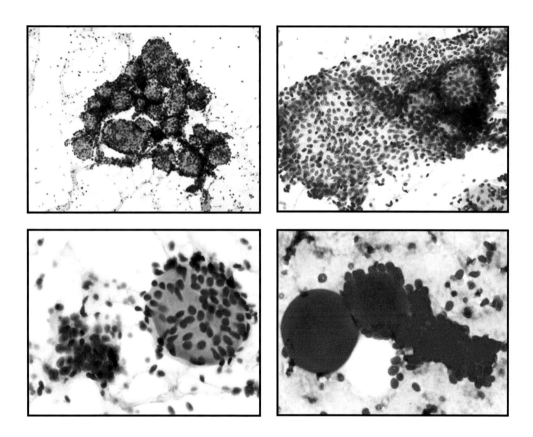

CASE

22

Clinical History

Fine needle aspiration of a left neck mass in an 83-year-old male.

Choose the Best Diagnosis

a. Adenoid cystic carcinoma

b. Carcinoma ex-pleomorphic adenoma

c. Cellular pleomorphic adenoma

d. Benign thyroid follicular epithelium

e. Adenomatoid nodule of thyroid

ANSWER AND BRIEF DISCUSSION

a. Adenoid Cystic Carcinoma

These are markedly cellular smears showing fragments of small basaloid-type cells with bland-appearing nuclei and a scant amount of cytoplasm. In addition, there are a large number of acellular spherules. Focally, these spherules are surrounded by the previously described basaloid cells. Although the exact anatomic location of this consultative case was not stated, it is almost certainly a salivary gland neoplasm.

If one looks only at the cellular material in this slide, one would be hesitant to make a diagnosis of a malignancy because the nuclei are very bland and contain few malignant features. The key to the diagnosis here are the acellular spherules with a bright magenta coloration on Diff-Quik and pale green refractile appearance on Papanicolaou stain, which are characteristic of adenoid cystic carcinoma.

References

1. Kapadia SB, Dusenbery D, Dekker A. Fine needle aspiration of pleomorphic adenoma and adenoid cystic carcinoma of salivary gland origin. *Acta Cytol*. 1997;41(2):487–492.
2. Nagel H, Hotze HJ, Laskawi R, Chilla R, Droese M. Cytologic diagnosis of adenoid cystic carcinoma of salivary glands. *Diagn Cytopathol*. 1999;20(6):358–366.

CASE

23

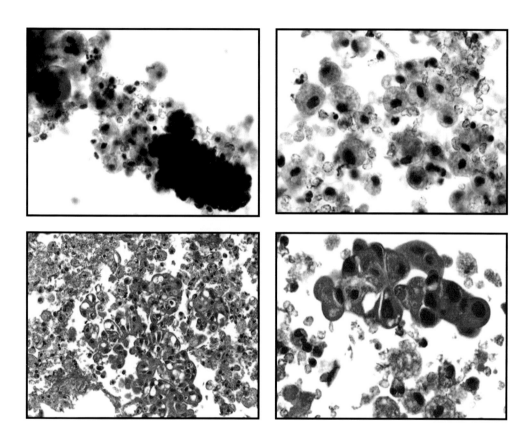

Ovarian cyst fluid aspirated from a 58-year-old female.

a. Benign follicular cyst of the ovary

b. Endometriosis

c. Teratoma

d. Adenocarcinoma

e. Lymphoma

ANSWER AND BRIEF DISCUSSION

d. Adenocarcinoma

The specimen contains numerous vacuolated cells, some appearing to be hemosiderin-laden macrophages, as well as scattered fragments of atypical epithelium, most evident on the cell block preparation.

When the cytospins are examined, they appear to be composed largely of vacuolated cells and many hemosiderin-laden macrophages. The presence of these vacuolated cells raises the possibility of a simple functional cyst; however, this woman is 58 years old and this ovarian cyst is quite large. Despite the patient's age, the presence of hemosiderin-laden macrophages in an ovarian cyst raises the possibility of endometriosis. However, in this case, no obvious benign endometrial-type epithelium and stroma is identified to make a definitive diagnosis of endometriosis. Instead, there are several fragments of markedly atypical epithelium on the cell block. These epithelial fragments are clearly glandular and have marked nuclear atypia consistent with an adenocarcinoma. Upon resection, this patient is found to have a well-differentiated endometrioid carcinoma of the ovary. Interestingly, the carcinoma appears to be arising in an endometriotic cyst.

References

1. Martinez-Onsurbe P, Ruiz Villaespesa A, Sanz Anquela JM, Valenzuela Ruiz PL. Aspiration cytology of 147 adnexal cysts with histologic correlation. *Acta Cytol.* 2001;45(6):941–947.
2. Mulvany NJ. Aspiration cytology of ovarian cysts and cystic neoplasms. A study of 235 aspirates. *Acta Cytol.* 1996;40(5):911–920.

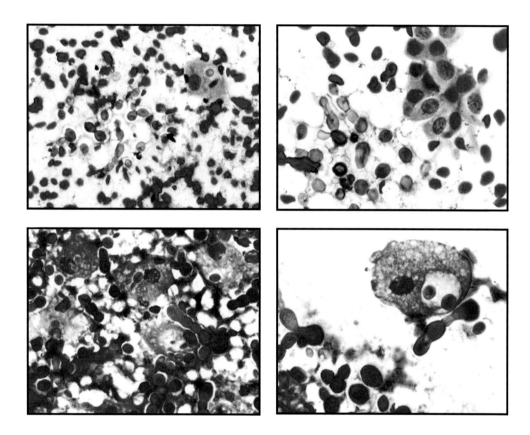

Clinical History

Transbronchial lung fine needle aspiration in a 30-year-old HIV+ male.

Choose the Best Diagnosis

    a. Histoplasmosis

    b. Cryptococcosis

    c. Candidiasis

    d. Blastomycosis

    e. Starch granules

ANSWER AND BRIEF DISCUSSION

b. Cryptococcosis

This specimen reveals large numbers of structures that are approximately 5 to 10 microns in diameter, have a peripheral clearing, and focally appear to be budding.

The morphologic appearance of these structures suggests that they are yeast. The extracellular location and the size rule out histoplasmosis. The round nature and the budding of these structures raise the possibility of blastomycosis. However, the yeast forms are too small and the budding appears to be predominantly narrow at the neck. Another feature of *Cryptococcus* is the variable sizes of the yeast forms. These features, along with the suggestion of a capsule around the yeast, are most consistent with cryptococcosis. Microbial cultures confirmed this morphologic impression. A mucicarmine stain is specific for the capsule of *Cryptococcus*.

References

1. Silverman JF. Inflammatory and neoplastic processes of the lung: differential diagnosis and pitfalls in FNA biopsies. *Diagn Cytopathol.* 1995;13(5):448–462.
2. Silverman JF, Johnsrude IS. Fine needle aspiration cytology of granulomatous cryptococcosis of the lung. *Acta Cytol.* 1985;29(2):157–161.

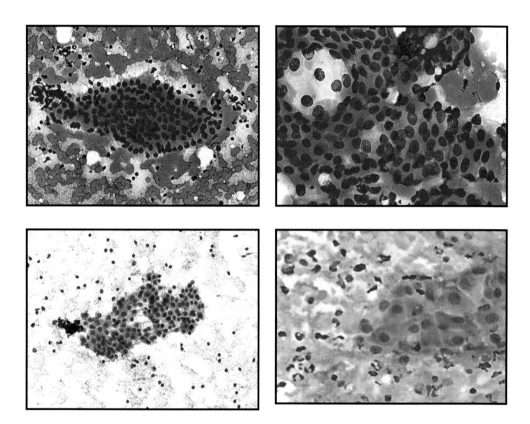

Clinical History

Fine needle aspiration of a parotid mass in a 52-year-old female.

Choose the Best Diagnosis

a. Retention cyst with squamous metaplasia

b. Lymphoepithelial cyst

c. Warthin tumor

d. Mucoepidermoid carcinoma (MEC)

e. Metastatic squamous cell carcinoma

ANSWER AND BRIEF DISCUSSION

c. Warthin Tumor

These slides contain a large amount of acellular proteinaceous material in the background as well as scattered individual lymphocytes and lymphoid tangles. In addition to these elements, there are scattered epithelial fragments present. These epithelial fragments contain large round nuclei with prominent central nucleoli and abundant granular cytoplasm, signifying oncocytic differentiation.

The presence of proteinaceous material and scattered lymphocytes raises the possibility that this is a cystic lesion, perhaps a simple retention cyst or (if this were an HIV+ individual) a benign lymphoepithelial cyst. However, the epithelial fragments that are present have the classic appearance of oncocytic cells. Thus, the combination of oncocytic epithelium along with a background of lymphocytes and proteinaceous debris suggests the diagnosis of Warthin tumor. Other cystic lesions that should be considered include MEC and metastatic squamous carcinoma; however, the atypia within the squamous epithelium in both these lesions is more pronounced than that seen in this lesion. The presence of focal oncocytic cells alone is not sufficient for a diagnosis of Warthin tumor because oncocytomas and focal oncocytic metaplasia can occur in lesions such as pleomorphic adenomas.

It is useful to remember the other name for a Warthin tumor, that is, a papillary cystadenoma lymphomatosum.

References

1. Parwani AV, Ali SZ. Diagnostic accuracy and pitfalls in fine-needle aspiration interpretation of warthin tumor. *Cancer.* 2003;99(3):166–171.
2. Mukunyadzi P. Review of fine-needle aspiration cytology of salivary gland neoplasms, with emphasis on differential diagnosis. *AJCP.* 2002;118(suppl):S100–S115.

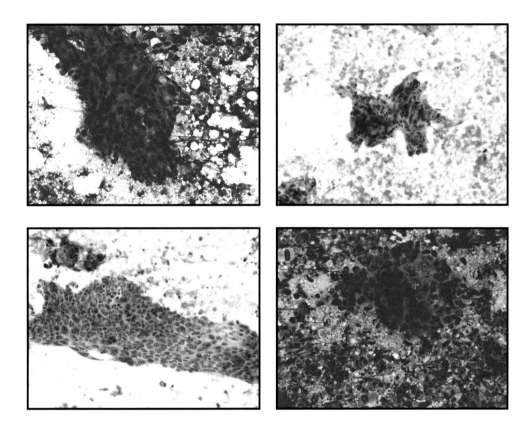

Clinical History

Lung fine needle aspiration in a 51-year-old female.

Choose the Best Diagnosis

a. Atypical bronchial epithelium

b. Carcinoma with bronchioloalveolar features

c. Small cell carcinoma

d. Metastatic adenocarcinoma, most consistent with colon primary

e. Carcinoid tumor

ANSWER AND BRIEF DISCUSSION

d. Metastatic Adenocarcinoma, Most Consistent With Colon Primary

These smears show numerous scattered moderately sized epithelial fragments. The fragments contain cells with large, pleomorphic oval-shaped nuclei with prominent nucleoli. There is marked disorganization within these fragments.

The epithelial fragments present here clearly represent a carcinoma due to their pleomorphism and disorganization. In areas, they have a columnar appearance with a prominent palisading of the nuclei and a moderate amount of apical cytoplasm. While this striking columnar appearance can be seen with some primary lung carcinomas, it is most consistent with a metastatic carcinoma from the gastrointestinal tract, which this patient had.

Reference

1. Cameron SEH, Andrade RS, Pambuccian SE. Endobronchial ultrasound-guided transbronchial needle aspiration cytology: a state of the art review. *Cytopathology*. 2010;21(1):6–26.

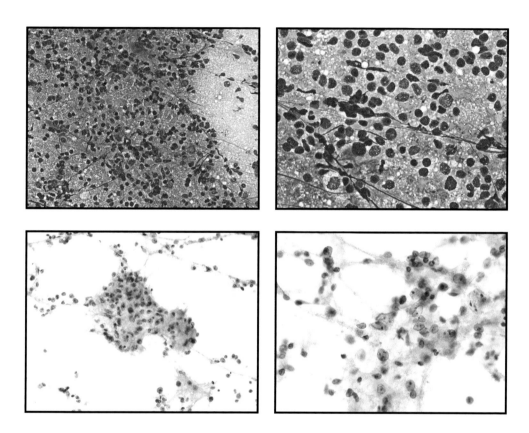

Clinical History

Fine needle aspiration of a frontal lobe brain mass in a 58-year-old male.

Choose the Best Diagnosis

    a. Metastatic small cell carcinoma

    b. High-grade glioma

    c. Granulomatous inflammation

    d. Large cell lymphoma

    e. Oligodendroglioma

ANSWER AND BRIEF DISCUSSION

d. Large Cell Lymphoma

This is a markedly cellular aspirate composed of small loosely cohesive irregular tissue fragments/aggregates and numerous single cells. The individual cells are predominantly naked nuclei or present as very high N/C ratio cells. The nuclei are larger than mature lymphocytes and focally have prominent nucleoli. A few reactive glial cells are also seen in the background.

At low power, the presence of large irregular and pleomorphic nuclei raised the possibility of glioblastoma multiforme. However, closer inspection of the individual cells suggest that they are likely lymphoid in origin. Another possibility based on the distinct single cell pattern is a metastatic small cell carcinoma; however, the chromatin does not appear neuroendocrine. An inflammatory lesion should be considered; however, the cellularity and relative monotonous population of cells argues against this. Flow cytometric immunophenotyping revealed a monoclonal B-cell phenotype, Kappa positive. There was also expression of the activation marker CD71. Taken together, the morphology and the immunophenotype suggest that this is a high-grade B-cell lymphoma.

References

1. Seliem RM, Assaad MW, Gorombey SJ, Moral LA, Kirkwood JR, Otis CN. Fine-needle aspiration biopsy of the central nervous system performed freehand under computed tomography guidance without stereotactic instrumentation. *Cancer*. 2003;99(5):277–284.
2. Silverman JF, Timmons RL, Leonard JR III, et al. Cytologic results of fine-needle aspiration biopsies of the central nervous system. *Cancer*. 1986;58(5):1117–1121.

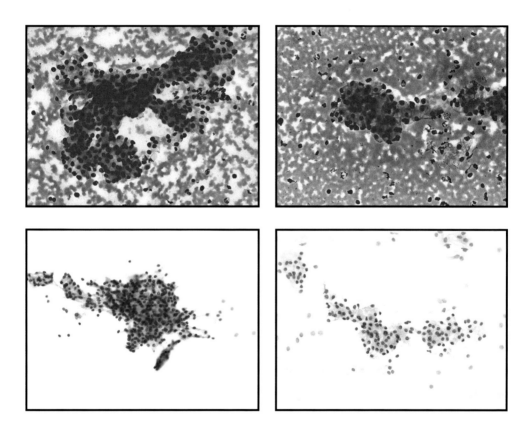

Fine needle aspiration of parotid gland in a 13-year-old girl.

a. Pleomorphic adenoma

b. Warthin tumor

c. Benign acinar tissue

d. Acinic cell carcinoma

e. Oncocytoma

ANSWER AND BRIEF DISCUSSION

d. Acinic Cell Carcinoma

The smears are cellular and show numerous cohesive tissue fragments with intact cells and a few scattered naked nuclei. The tumor cells are large and have abundant cytoplasm that ranges from clear to coarsely granular. The nuclei are round and fairly regular in size. Some of the cells have prominent nucleoli. The background is vaguely granular.

The cytomorphologic features are consistent with acinic cell carcinoma. Acinic cell carcinoma cells often depict small uniform nuclei and can be confused with benign acinar tissue. The lack of a lobulated "bunch of grapes"-like appearance, the cellularity of the specimen, and the presence of naked nuclei and cellular debris suggest against benign tissue. The naked nuclei frequently seen associated with the tissue fragment can be mistaken for lymphocytes (leading to an incorrect diagnosis of Warthin tumor). Oncocytic neoplasms should also be considered, but the quality of the cytoplasm is more consistent with the zymogen granules of acinic cells than the finely granular cytoplasm typical of oncocytes.

References

1. Nagel H, Laskawi R, Buter JJ, Schroder M, Chilla R, Droese M. Cytologic diagnosis of acinic-cell carcinoma of salivary glands. *Diagn Cytopathol*. 1997;16(5):402–412.
2. Stewart CJ, MacKenzie K, McGarry GW, Mowat A. Fine-needle aspiration cytology of salivary gland: a review of 341 cases. *Diagn Cytopathol*. 2000;22(3):139–146.

CASE

29

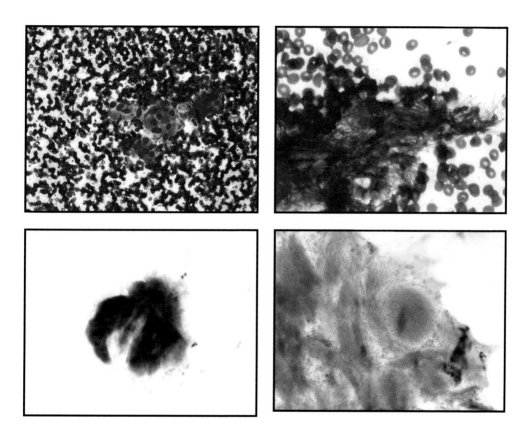

Clinical History

Fine needle aspiration (FNA) of a 4-cm prepatellar mass in a 51-year-old man. The patient has a history of gout that involved his great toe but never his knee.

Choose the Best Diagnosis

    a. Amyloid nodule

    b. Findings consistent with gout

    c. Inflammatory myofibroblastic tumor

    d. Atypical cells worrisome for sarcoma

    e. Actinomyces with abscess formation

ANSWER AND BRIEF DISCUSSION

b. Findings Consistent With Gout

The smears show scattered mononuclear and multinucleated histiocytes associated with aggregates of needle-shaped crystals. Rare fibroblasts and inflammatory cells are also identified.

The findings are compatible with a gouty tophus. Several patients have been reported in whom a gouty tophus was so large that it closely mimicked a soft tissue neoplasm. In such cases, FNA may be warranted to avoid unnecessary surgery. Amyloid is another extracellular material that can accumulate in amounts that can clinically simulate a neoplasm. Amyloid deposits are irregular fragments with well-delineated edges that may be scalloped or straight.

References

1. Bhadani PP, Sah SP, Sen R, Singh RK. Diagnostic value of fine needle aspiration cytology in gouty tophi: a report of 7 cases. *Acta Cytol.* 2006;50(1):101–104.
2. Nicol KK, Ward WG, Pike EJ, Geisinger KR, Cappellari JO, Kilpatrick SE. Fine-needle aspiration biopsy of gouty tophi: lessons in cost-effective patient management. *Diagn Cytopathol.* 1997;17(1):30–35.

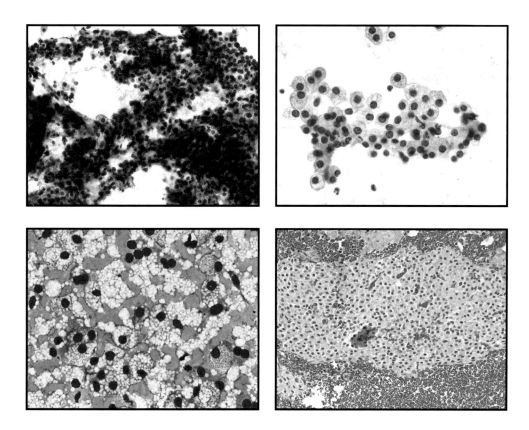

Clinical History

Fine needle aspiration (FNA) of a 2.8-cm adrenal mass in a 75-year-old woman.

Choose the Best Diagnosis

a. Benign cyst fluid

b. Angiomyolipoma

c. Pheochromocytoma

d. Metastatic adenocarcinoma

e. Adrenal cortical neoplasm

ANSWER AND BRIEF DISCUSSION

e. Adrenal Cortical Neoplasm

This is a cellular specimen containing a monotonous population of neoplastic cells. The cells are present in discohesive fragments, clusters, and individual cells. In some fields, naked nuclei can be identified. The cells have distinct borders and significant cytoplasmic vacuolization. Prominent nucleoli are not seen. On the cell block, the cells are organized in a solid/trabecular growth pattern, and no gland formation is appreciated. Neither mitotic figures nor necrosis is identified.

Adrenal cortical neoplasms arise from adrenal cortical tissue and are composed of cells resembling any of the three layers: zona glomerulosa, zona fasciculata, and zone reticularis. Adrenal cortical adenomas are well circumscribed and are often identified incidentally; most are nonfunctional. Differentiating an adrenal cortical adenoma from an adrenal cortical carcinoma is not possible on FNA alone, though it is extremely rare for small (<5 cm) lesions to be carcinomas. In this case, there are no features suggesting a metastatic adenocarcinoma, such as gland formation or the presence of mucin, and metastases are often present bilaterally, with the lung being the most common primary site. Given the close proximity of the kidney to the adrenal gland, renal cell carcinoma should always be excluded, given the overlap of several cytomorphologic features. However, the absence of distinct nucleoli in this case does not favor a renal cell carcinoma. When a cell block is available, adrenal cortical neoplasms may demonstrate immunoreactivity with inhibin, Melan-A, SF-1, and synaptophysin, but are negative for chromogranin and S-100 protein.

References

1. Lloyd RV. Adrenal cortical tumors, pheochromocytomas and paragangliomas. *Mod Pathol.* 2011;24(suppl 2):S58–S65.
2. Stelow EB, Debol SM, Stanley MW, Mallery S, Lai R, Bardales RH. Sampling of the adrenal glands by endoscopic ultrasound-guided fine-needle aspiration. *Diagn Cytopathol.* 2005;33(1):26–30.

CASE

31

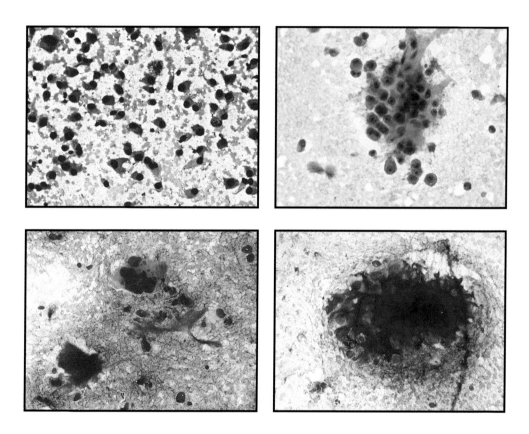

Clinical History

Fine needle aspiration (FNA) of a right distal femur lesion in a 22-year-old female.

Choose the Best Diagnosis

    a. Metastatic renal cell carcinoma

    b. Metastatic melanoma

    c. Giant cell tumor of bone

    d. Plasmablastic lymphoma

    e. Osteosarcoma

ANSWER AND BRIEF DISCUSSION

e. Osteosarcoma

At low power, the smears consist of scattered discohesive, predominantly plasmacytoid cells. The cytoplasm is basophilic and finely vacuolated. The Papanicolaou stain demonstrates the presence of prominent nucleoli. Overall, there is striking nuclear pleomorphism, and some multinucleated cells can be identified. The Diff-Quik stain reveals magenta-colored matrix material, which has a dense look in some areas; this is disorganized, malignant osteoid that is a defining feature of osteoblastic osteosarcoma. This feature, coupled with the clinical scenario, favors this entity over the other choices.

Osteoblastic osteosarcoma comprises 50% of conventional osteosarcomas, which in turn account for 90% of all osteosarcomas. It is unclear whether the osteoblastic subtype has any prognostic significance. In one series, the average patient age was 17 years old, with a 4:3 male to female ratio. In an older patient, metastatic tumors to the bone are more common than primary bone tumors, and these are often easily diagnosed on FNA. Distinguishing primary bone tumors on FNA is much more challenging, and definitive diagnosis often relies heavily upon histological and radiological examination.

References

1. Sathiyamoorthy S, Ali SZ. Osteoblastic osteosarcoma: cytomorphologic characteristics and differential diagnosis on fine-needle aspiration. *Acta Cytol.* 2012;56(5):481–486.
2. White VA, Fanning CV, Ayala AG, Raymond AK, Carrasco CH, Murray JA. Osteosarcoma and the role of fine needle aspiration. A study of 51 cases. *Cancer.* 1988;62(6):1238–1246.

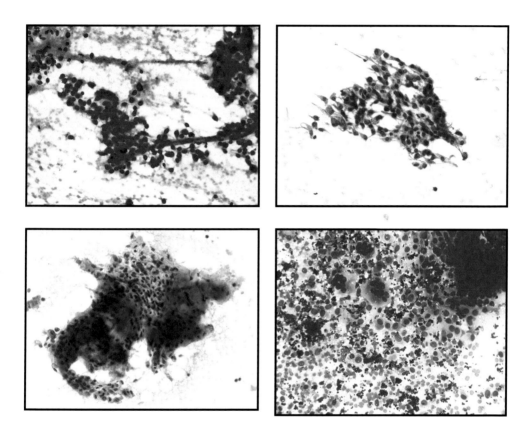

Clinical History

Fine needle aspiration of a 5.2-cm posterior right knee mass in a 39-year-old woman.

Choose the Best Diagnosis

    a. Giant cell tumor of tendon sheath

    b. Chondroblastoma

    c. Metastatic adenocarcinoma

    d. Metastatic melanoma

    e. Pigmented villonodular synovitis (PVNS)

ANSWER AND BRIEF DISCUSSION

e. Pigmented Villonodular Synovitis (PVNS)

The lesion consists primarily of round and spindled cells with bland, eccentrically placed nuclei. The cytoplasm is granular and occasionally vacuolated. The cells exist in fragments as well as single cells. Multinucleated giant cells are also identified, containing the same regular, round, and bland nuclei of the surrounding single cells. Papanicolaou stain preparations demonstrate a green-brown cytoplasmic pigment. Some cellular fragments are intimately associated with matrix material or vessels.

PVNS arises from the synovial lining of joints and generally presents as a unilateral knee mass. While its name may be misleading, PVNS is thought to be a neoplastic process comprising multinuclear giant cells and accompanying mononuclear cells with many morphological similarities to a giant cell tumor of the tendon sheath. The neoplastic cells are of histiocytic origin, are immunoreactive for CD68, and often contain pigment. While PVNS is considered a benign neoplasm, it can be locally aggressive and appear to erode into the underlying bone; local recurrence is not uncommon.

References

1. Dorwant RH, Genant HK, Johnston WH, Morris JM. Pigmented villonodular synovitis of synovial joints: clinical, pathologic, and radiologic features. *Am J of Roent.* 1984;143(4):877–885.
2. Khalbuss WE, Parwani AV. Cytopathology of Soft Tissue and Bone Lesions Containing Giant Cells. *Cytopathology of Soft Tissue and Bone Lesions, Essentials in Cytopathology.* 2011;11–40.

CASE

33

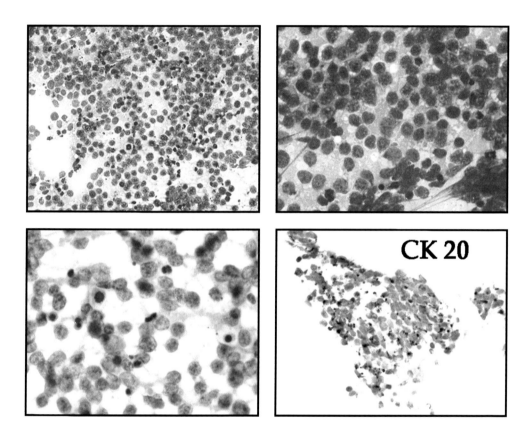

Clinical History

Fine needle aspiration of a left forearm mass in a 54-year-old woman.

Choose the Best Diagnosis

a. High-grade lymphoma

b. Chondroid syringoma

c. Epidermal inclusion cyst with reactive atypia

d. Merkel cell carcinoma (MCC)

e. Melanoma

ANSWER AND BRIEF DISCUSSION

d. Merkel Cell Carcinoma (MCC)

The cellular aspirates show a monotonous population of overtly malignant cells. The cells show increased N/C ratios with very little cytoplasm and have even, finely granular chromatin. The cells are loosely cohesive, and numerous mitotic figures and apoptotic figures are present. The CK-20 immunostain shows perinuclear "dotlike" positivity.

The described cytomorphologic features and immunoprofile are diagnostic of MCC. Other considerations based on the morphology would include high-grade lymphoma and metastasis from a primary lung small cell carcinoma. MCC is a rare, aggressive cutaneous malignancy that predominates in older Caucasians. The tumor is thought to arise from Merkel cells, which are located in the basal layer of the epidermis and may function in mechanoreception. MCC can be difficult to distinguish from other "small blue cell" neoplasms, and as such, immunohistochemical stains should be utilized. The perinuclear dot-like positivity observed in this case is typical of MCC.

References

1. al-Kaisi NK. Fine-needle aspiration cytology of a metastatic Merkel-cell carcinoma. *Diagn Cytopathol*. 1991;7(2):184–188.
2. Bechert CJ, Schnadig V, Nawgiri R. The Merkel cell carcinoma challenge: a review from the fine needle aspiration service. *Cancer Cytopathol*. 2013;121(4):179–188.

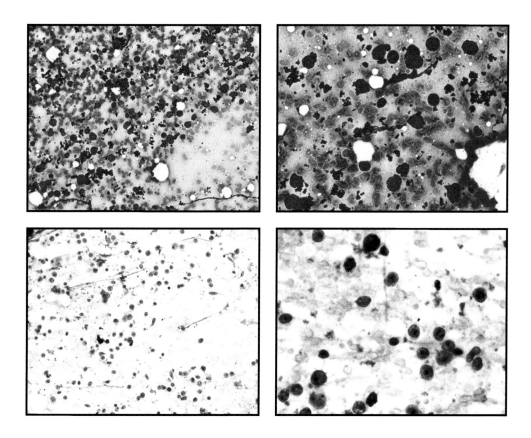

Clinical History

Fine needle aspiration of a retroperitoneal lymph node in a 77-year-old woman with abdominal lymphadenopathy and a mass involving the head of the pancreas.

Choose the Best Diagnosis

a. Carcinoma with signet ring cell features

b. Diffuse large B-cell lymphoma

c. Small cell carcinoma

d. Acinar cell carcinoma

e. Chronic pancreatitis

ANSWER AND BRIEF DISCUSSION

b. Diffuse Large B-Cell Lymphoma

The smears are moderately cellular and show a monomorphic population of atypical large lymphoid cells. The nuclei have moderate variation in shape with clumped and cleared chromatin patterns. Many of the cells have prominent nucleoli. Very little cytoplasm is discernible.

The cytomorphologic features are consistent with diffuse large B-cell lymphoma. The differential includes both poorly differentiated carcinoma and melanoma. The presence of true cohesion and tissue fragments in carcinomas and pigment granules in melanomas can be helpful distinguishing features. Subsequent tissue studies confirmed the cytologic diagnosis.

References

1. Nayer H, Weir EG, Sheth S, Ali SZ. Primary pancreatic lymphomas: a cytopathologic analysis of a rare malignancy. *Cancer*. 2004;102(5):315–321.
2. Volmar KE, Routbort MJ, Jones CK, Xie HB. Primary pancreatic lymphoma evaluated by fine-needle aspiration: findings in 14 cases. *AJCP*. 2004;121(6):898–903.

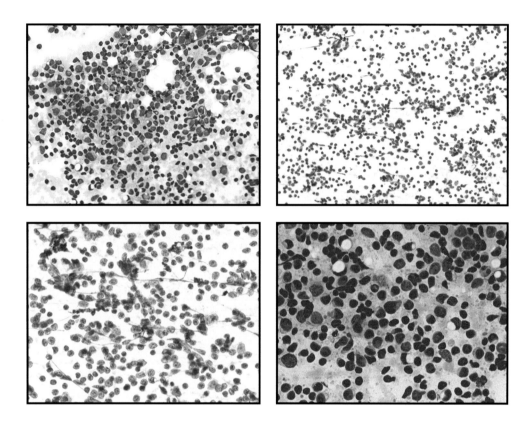

Clinical History

Fine needle aspiration of a cervical lymph node in a 43-year-old male.

Choose the Best Diagnosis

    a. Follicular hyperplasia

    b. Hodgkin lymphoma

    c. Malignant lymphoma, low-grade follicular cell type

    d. Malignant lymphoma, large B-cell type

    e. Metastatic small cell carcinoma

ANSWER AND BRIEF DISCUSSION

c. Malignant Lymphoma, Low-Grade Follicular Cell Type

Smears reveal a moderately cellular specimen composed predominantly of individual lymphoid cells. Although there is some pleomorphism in this population, the majority of the cells appear to be composed of intermediate-sized cells with nuclear membrane abnormalities.

One might consider a reactive process in this node, but the monotony among the intermediate-sized population, along with the nuclear membrane abnormalities, argues that this is a lymphoproliferative disorder. Immunophenotyping by flow cytometry revealed an abnormal population of B cells that demonstrates lambda light chain restriction and positivity for CD19, CD20, and CD10. This abnormal population was negative for CD5. The combination of this morphology and immunophenotype is suggestive of a malignant lymphoma, B-cell type, possibly of follicular center cell origin. The lack of high-grade morphologic features and only weak expression of the activation marker CD71 argue that this is a low-grade lymphoma.

Reference

1. Young NA. Grading follicular lymphoma on fine-needle aspiration specimens—a practical approach. *Cancer.* 2006;108(1):1–9.

CASE

36

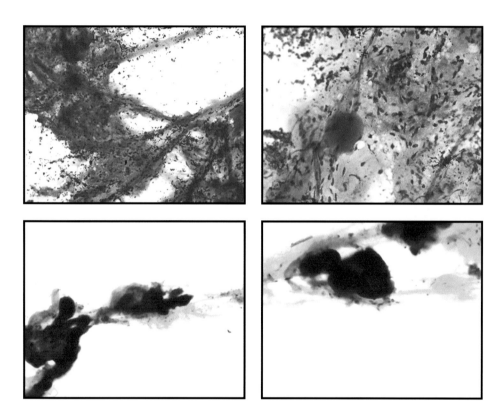

Clinical History

A 72-year-old woman presents with pain in her left shoulder and is found to have a 3.0-cm soft-tissue mass. Radiographic studies show that the lesion involved muscle and soft tissue in the subscapular region and appeared infiltrative at its margins. She has no previous history of malignancy and is otherwise in good health.

Choose the Best Diagnosis

a. Nodular fasciitis

b. Myxoid liposarcoma

c. Elastofibroma

d. Ischemic fasciitis

e. Lipoma

ANSWER AND BRIEF DISCUSSION

c. Elastofibroma

The smears are moderately cellular and show bland spindle cells with acellular collagen bundles and looser myxoid areas in the background. Additionally, curious linear and globular structures were present on the Diff-Quik-stained material. Atypia and necrosis were not present.

The cytologic findings are consistent with elastofibroma dorsi (EFD). EFD is probably a reactive condition that has distinct clinical and radiographic features. It usually occurs in elderly females near the inferior margin of the scapula. The cytomorphologic features have been described and include moderately cellular smears consisting of bland spindled cells, acellular collagen, and distinct linear (termed "braided hair" and "fern leaf") and globular elastic fibers. Histologic follow-up confirmed the cytologic diagnosis.

References

1. Domanski HA. Fine-needle aspiration of ganglioneuroma. *Diagn Cytopathol.* 2005;32(6):363–366.
2. Domanski HA. Elastic fibers in elastofibroma dorsi by fine-needle aspiration. *Diagn Cytopathol.* 2013;42(7):609–611.

CASE

37

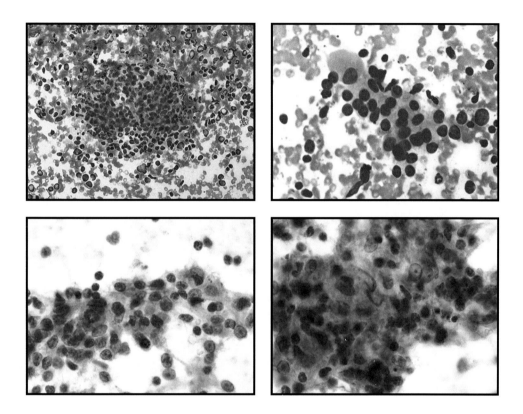

Clinical History

A 41-year-old woman presents with a sensation of "fullness" in her neck for the past few years. She also feels "nervous and jittery" for several days at a time, reports occasional insomnia, and has frequent bowel movements (5–7 times a day). She denies heat intolerance. Ultrasound-guided fine needle aspiration of thyroid.

Choose the Best Diagnosis

a. Adenomatoid nodule

b. Suspicious for a follicular neoplasm

c. Papillary carcinoma

d. Medullary carcinoma

e. Lymphocytic thyroiditis

ANSWER AND BRIEF DISCUSSION

e. Lymphocytic Thyroiditis

The smears display numerous cellular aggregates and single cells seen at low power. High power reveals a mixed lymphocytic population scattered among Hurthle cells. The Hurthle cells have large round nuclei, prominent nucleoli, abundant cytoplasm, and rare mitotic figures.

The abundant discohesive lymphocytic population is highly suggestive of an inflammatory lesion; one should be cautious about diagnosing carcinoma based on atypia seen with a prominent inflammatory background. The colloid to epithelium ratio would be much higher in an adenomatoid nodule. In follicular neoplasms, one would find more epithelial cells arranged in microfollicles without the inflammatory component seen here. Finally, medullary carcinomas typically have an abundance of cells with neuroendocrine ("salt-and-pepper") nuclei, occasional plasmacytoid and spindled features, and associated amyloid. Subsequent thyroidectomy showed a multinodular hyperplasia with chronic lymphocytic thyroiditis (Hashimoto thyroiditis).

References

1. Harvey AM, Truong LD, Mody DR. Diagnostic pitfalls of hashimoto's/lymphocytic thyroiditis on fine-needle aspirations and strategies to avoid overdiagnosis. *Acta Cytol*. 2012;56(4):352–360.
2. Baloch ZW, Cibas ES, Clark DP, et al. The national cancer institute thyroid fine needle aspiration state of the science conference: a summation. *CytoJournal*. 2008;5(1):6.

CASE

38

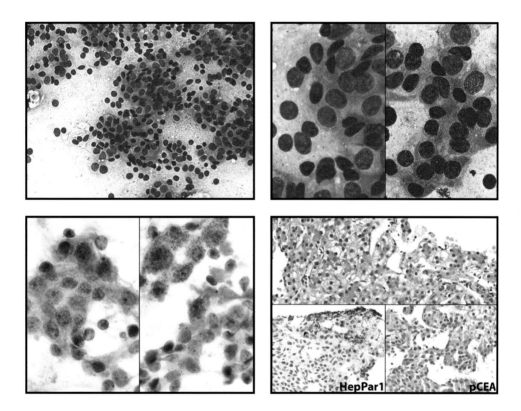

Clinical History

A 23-month-old girl presents with a 1-week history of fussiness, decreased oral intake, occasional nonbloody, nonbilious emesis, and increasing complaints of pain. Abdominal CT reveals a 14-cm liver mass. Thoracic CT reveals multiple small lung nodules measuring up to 5 mm in maximum diameter. Ultrasound-guided fine needle aspiration of liver.

Choose the Best Diagnosis

    a. Focal nodular hyperplasia

    b. Hepatic adenoma

    c. Hepatoblastoma

    d. Hepatocellular carcinoma (HCC)

    e. Lymphoma

ANSWER AND BRIEF DISCUSSION

c. Hepatoblastoma

The specimen is very cellular and consists of numerous tissue fragments with scattered single cells in the background. There are two cytologically distinct cell populations. The cells of one population have large round nuclei with a single prominent nucleolus, numerous cytoplasmic granules, and a high N/C ratio. The cells of the second population are smaller, have an even higher N/C ratio, and have hyperchromatic elongated nuclei without nucleoli. Within each population, the cells are relatively uniform (ie, pleomorphism is not significant). The tissue core shows vaguely trabecular architecture, and the cells are immunoreactive for HepPar1.

Hepatoblastoma is the most common hepatic malignancy in the pediatric population. Hepatoblastomas typically fall into two categories: epithelial and mixed epithelial-mesenchymal. The epithelial component is composed of varying proportions of cells having features described as embryonal (as seen in the smaller cells of this case) or fetal (seen in the larger cells of this case). Other less common variants include anaplastic small cell and macrotrabecular. An important entity to exclude in the differential diagnosis is HCC. Features that favor hepatoblastoma include metaplastic elements (eg, osteoid) and extramedullary hematopoiesis. Features that suggest HCC include marked pleomorphism and giant cells.

References

1. Wakely PE Jr, Silverman JF, Geisinger KR, Frable WJ. Fine needle aspiration biopsy cytology of hepatoblastoma. *Mod Pathol.* 1990;3(6):688–693.
2. Weir EG, Ali SZ. Hepatoblastoma: cytomorphologic characteristics in serous cavity fluids. *Cancer.* 2002;96(5):267–274.

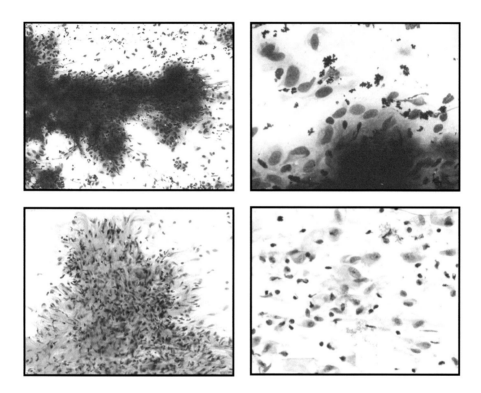

Clinical History

Fine needle aspiration of a 1.8-cm chest wall mass in a 35-year-old man. He states the mass has been present for 6 months with no apparent change in size. The lesion evolved rapidly after the patient was struck by a batted ball in a softball game. The lesion causes no symptoms but is slightly tender to palpation. Imaging studies reveal a well-demarcated soft-tissue mass that does not involve the adjacent rib.

Choose the Best Diagnosis

a. Malignant fibrohistiocytic tumor

b. Myxoid liposarcoma

c. Nodular fasciitis (NF)

d. Proliferative myositis

e. Chondrosarcoma

ANSWER AND BRIEF DISCUSSION

c. Nodular Fasciitis (NF)

The smears are highly cellular and are composed of single cells, tissue fragments, and loose aggregates in a metachromatic myxoid background. The tissue fragments are arranged haphazardly, imparting a "tissue culture" look. The cellular contours are variable. Some cells are spindled and others have more of an ovoid shape. The nuclei are round to oval with smooth contours and distinct small nucleoli.

The described features in conjunction with the clinical history are diagnostic of NF. The key in this case is to recognize the reactive/reparative look and not incorrectly classify as a sarcoma. NF is an important entity to be familiar with as it can be mistaken for a malignant process. Although its nature (neoplastic vs. reactive) is debatable, its behavior is benign.

References

1. Dahl I, Akerman M. Nodular fasciitis a correlative cytologic and histologic study of 13 cases. *Acta Cytol.* 1981;25(3):215–223.
2. Stanley MW, Skoog L, Tani EM, Horwitz CA. Nodular fasciitis: spontaneous resolution following diagnosis by fine-needle aspiration. *Diagn Cytopathol.* 1993;9(3):322–324.

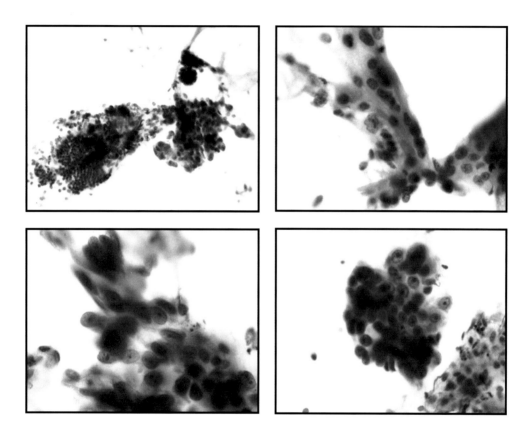

Clinical History

Pancreatic duct brushing in a 77-year-old black female.

Choose the Best Diagnosis

a. Reactive ductal epithelium

b. Intraductal papillary mucinous neoplasm

c. Adenocarcinoma

d. Pancreatic neuroendocrine tumor

e. Solid pseudopapillary neoplasm

ANSWER AND BRIEF DISCUSSION

c. Adenocarcinoma

These cellular images contain a variety of cell types including normal ductal epithelium as well as scattered irregular tissue fragments containing cells with markedly enlarged nuclei, nuclear pleomorphism, and prominent nucleoli.

It is important to act conservatively when dealing with focal atypia within an otherwise normal biliary tract or pancreatic duct brushing. Often these patients present with jaundice, and a stent is placed that can produce squamous metaplasia with marked reactive atypia. However in this case, there appear to be two distinct populations of cells, one with a perfectly benign, honeycomb appearance and a second population of markedly atypical cells with nuclear enlargement and pleomorphism. In this case, a diagnosis of adenocarcinoma is relatively straightforward. While this is most likely a pancreatic adenocarcinoma based on the clinical information given, a high-grade extrahepatic cholangiocarcinoma might appear similar.

Reference

1. Bellizzi AM, Stelow EB. Pancreatic cytopathology: a practical approach and review. *Arch Pathol Lab Med.* 2009;133(3):388–404.

CASE

41

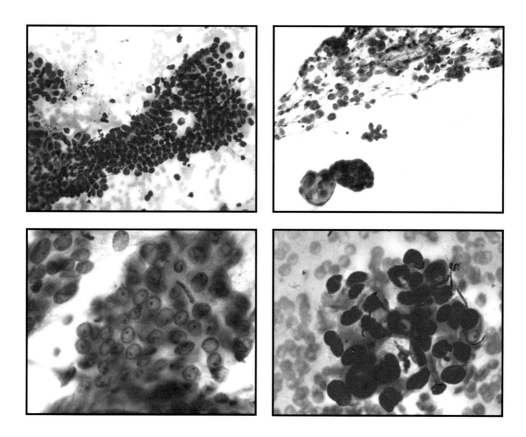

Clinical History

An ultrasound-guided fine needle aspiration of a lung mass in a 58-year-old white male.

Choose the Best Diagnosis

a. Adenocarcinoma with bronchioloalveolar features

b. Mesothelioma

c. Metastatic papillary renal cell carcinoma

d. Squamous cell carcinoma

e. Metastatic malignant melanoma

ANSWER AND BRIEF DISCUSSION

a. Adenocarcinoma With Bronchioloalveolar Features

This is a markedly cellular specimen containing large atypical epithelial fragments. The cells within these fragments contain enlarged nuclei with prominent grooves and occasional intranuclear inclusions.

This is clearly an adenocarcinoma, non-small cell type. It has some interesting features that include nuclear grooves and inclusions. In this setting, it would be important to exclude a metastatic papillary carcinoma of the thyroid gland, which could be done by thyroglobulin staining or a serum thyroglobulin level. Also, the patient would most likely have a thyroid nodule and cervical adenopathy. A primary lung tumor that can often display intranuclear inclusions is an adenocarcinoma with bronchioloalveolar features. Interestingly, a thyroid transcription factor-1 immunohistochemical stain would not be helpful in making this distinction because both thyroid carcinomas and primary lung carcinomas are positive for this transcription factor. However, a thyroglobulin could have made this distinction. An infiltrating moderately differentiated adenocarcinoma with focal bronchioloalveolar features was found on resection.

References

1. Atkins KA. The diagnosis of bronchioloalveolar carcinoma by cytologic means. *AJCP*. 2004;122(1):14–16.
2. Auger M, Katz RL, Johnston DA. Differentiating cytological features of bronchioloalveolar carcinoma from adenocarcinoma of the lung in fine-needle aspirations: a statistical analysis of 27 cases. *Diagn Cytopathol*. 1997;16(3):253–257.

CASE

42

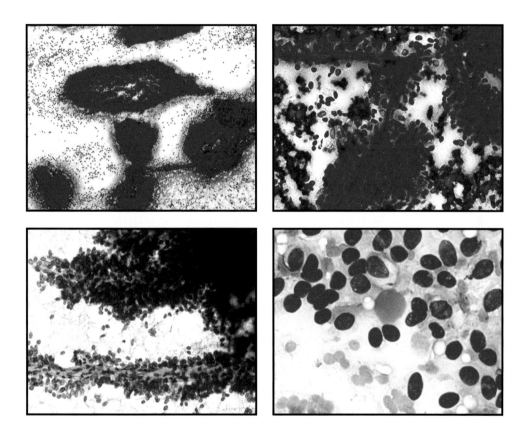

Clinical History

Endoscopic ultrasound-guided fine needle aspiration of a well-circumscribed, partially cystic 4-cm pancreatic mass in a 22-year-old woman.

Choose the Best Diagnosis

    a. Pancreatoblastoma

    b. Solid pseudopapillary neoplasm (SPN)

    c. Acinar cell carcinoma

    d. Pancreatic neuroendocrine tumor (PanNET)

    e. Ductal adenocarcinoma

ANSWER AND BRIEF DISCUSSION

b. Solid Pseudopapillary Neoplasm (SPN)

The aspirates are cellular and contain branching fibrovascular cores lined by multiple layers of relatively uniform tumor cells. The nuclei are round to oval with evenly distributed chromatin and discernible small nucleoli. Scattered hyaline globules are associated with the tumor cells.

SPN of the pancreas is a rare low-grade tumor that typically affects young women. This tumor should be suspected in any young female with a partially cystic pancreatic mass. Hyaline globules that are either intracellular or extracellular are characteristic and are very unusual in other primary pancreatic neoplasms. This tumor has substantial cytomorphologic overlap with PanNET. Immunohistochemical stains are useful in this distinction, with SPN showing reactivity for CD10, CD99, and beta-catenin. The histogenesis of SPN has been debated, but ultrastructural and immunohistochemical evidence supports an origin from a primitive pancreatic epithelial cell with capacity for dual (exocrine and endocrine) differentiation. The treatment is surgical and the prognosis is excellent.

References

1. Bardales RH, Centeno B, Mallery JS, et al. Endoscopic ultrasound-guided fine-needle aspiration cytology diagnosis of solid-pseudopapillary tumor of the pancreas: a rare neoplasm of elusive origin but characteristic cytomorphologic features. *AJCP*. 2004;121(5):654–662.
2. Pettinato G, Di Vizio D, Manivel JC, Pambuccian SE, Somma P, Insabato L. Solid-pseudopapillary tumor of the pancreas: a neoplasm with distinct and highly characteristic cytological features. *Diagn Cytopathol*. 2002;27(6):325–334.

CASE

43

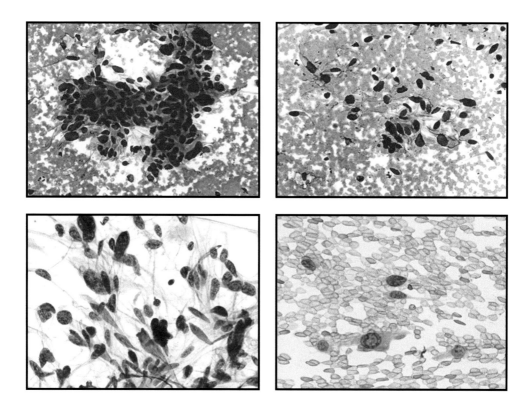

Fine needle aspiration of a scrotal mass in a 53-year-old man.

    a. High-grade sarcoma

    b. Poorly differentiated carcinoma

    c. Malignant mesothelioma

    d. Seminoma

    e. Large B-cell lymphoma

ANSWER AND BRIEF DISCUSSION

a. High-Grade Sarcoma

The aspirate contains fragments and single markedly atypical cells. The cells have predominantly spindled nuclei with a few that are more rounded. The nuclei are extremely pleomorphic. The chromatin is dense and granular. The cytoplasm is paler with a fibrillar quality.

The features are certainly diagnostic of malignancy. The cytomorphology is most consistent with a high-grade sarcoma. The lack of cohesion supports a nonepithelial origin of the tumor cells. Mesotheliomas would typically display more cohesive, rounder (epithelioid) cells. This individual had a history of a high-grade leiomyosarcoma of the pelvis. The case was signed out as consistent with recurrent leiomyosarcoma.

Reference

1. Domanski HA, Akerman H, Rissler P, Gustafson P. Fine-needle aspiration of soft tissue leiomyosarcoma: an analysis of the most common cytologic findings and the value of ancillary techniques. *Diagn Cytopathol*. 2006;34(9):597–604.

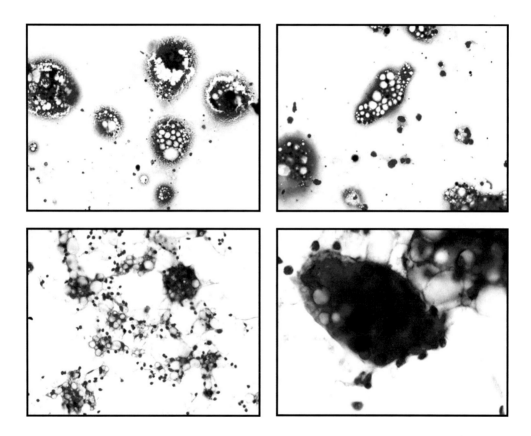

Clinical History

Fine needle aspiration (FNA) of an axillary mass in a 74-year-old woman.

Choose the Best Diagnosis

    a. Silicone lymphadenopathy

    b. Liposarcoma

    c. Metastatic breast carcinoma

    d. Atypical mycobacterium infection

    e. Hibernoma

ANSWER AND BRIEF DISCUSSION

a. Silicone Lymphadenopathy

The aspirates show numerous multinucleated giant cells with large round empty spaces and associated lymphocytes. The macrophage (shown here) contains linear magenta inclusions arranged around one of its nuclei. Necrosis is not present.

The findings are consistent with silicone lymphadenopathy. Clinically, this patient had a failing silicone breast implant at the time of FNA. The linear magenta inclusions mentioned here in the high-power image are suggestive of an "asteroid body" that can be seen in silicone reactions. Fat necrosis and subareolar abscess can produce similar findings with multinucleated giant cells. Fat necrosis tends to have smaller vacuoles, and subareolar abscess classically has ingested squamous cells in the cytoplasm of the histiocytes.

References

1. Tabatowski K, Elson CE, Johnston WW. Silicone lymphadenopathy in a patient with a mammary prosthesis. Fine needle aspiration cytology, histology and analytical electron microscopy. *Acta Cytol*. 1990;34(1):10–14.
2. Tabatowski K, Sammarco GJ. Fine needle aspiration cytology of silicone lymphadenopathy in a patient with an artificial joint. A case report. *Acta Cytol*. 1992;36(4):529–532.

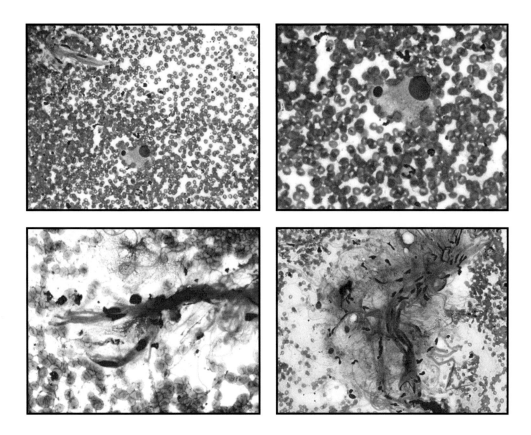

Clinical History

Fine needle aspiration of a 10-cm retroperitoneal mass in a 22-year-old man.

Choose the Best Diagnosis

 a. Liposarcoma

 b. Malignant peripheral nerve sheath tumor (MPNST)

 c. Neuroblastoma with favorable features

 d. Ganglioneuroma

 e. Malignant melanoma

ANSWER AND BRIEF DISCUSSION

d. Ganglioneuroma

The aspirates show bland spindled cells with wavy, pointed nuclei embedded in a metachromatic stroma. Occasionally, mature ganglion cells with macronucleoli are also present. Necrosis and significant atypia are not identified.

The combination of mature nerve elements and ganglion cells in a single tumor is diagnostic of ganglioneuroma. Although ganglion cells are a favorable prognostic finding in neuroblastoma, there are no cytologic features in this case to suggest neuroblastoma. Liposarcoma should be considered because of the location, but again there is no cytologic support for this diagnosis. MPNST would be expected to show neural features as well as overt features of malignancy (necrosis, severe atypia, etc.).

References

1. Domanski HA. Fine-needle aspiration of ganglioneuroma. *Diagn Cytopathol.* 2005;32(6):363–366.
2. Yen H, Cobb CJ. Retroperitoneal ganglioneuroma: a report of diagnosis by fine-needle aspiration cytology. *Diagn Cytopathol.* 1998;19(5):385–387.

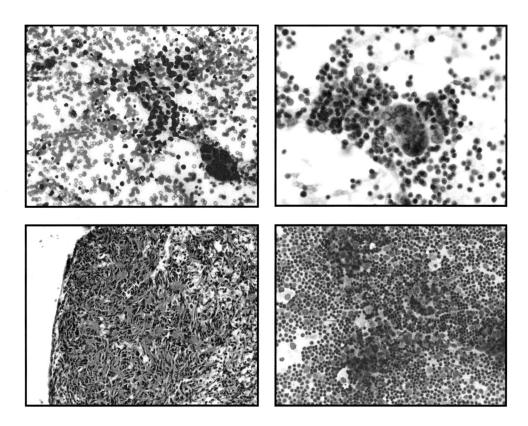

Clinical History

Fine needle aspiration of an anterior mediastinal mass in a 49-year-old female.

Choose the Best Diagnosis

a. Thymoma

b. Lymphoma

c. Teratoma

d. Small cell carcinoma

e. Carcinoid

ANSWER AND BRIEF DISCUSSION

a. Thymoma

The slides reveal an abundant polymorphous lymphoid population as well as aggregates of epithelioid cells. While the differential diagnosis of an anterior mediastinal mass includes lymphoma, the lymphoid cells present here are generally small and the population is somewhat polymorphous. The presence of epithelioid cells intermixed with this lymphoid population suggests that this may represent a thymoma. In this case, immunophenotyping displayed immature T cells, with a range of expression of CD3, dim CD10 expression, and positivity for CD1a, CD4, CD8, and CD5. Taken together, these findings are consistent with a thymoma.

Reference

1. Ali SZ, Erozan YS. Thymoma. Cytopathologic features and differential diagnosis on fine needle aspiration. *Acta Cytol.* 1998;42(4):845–854.

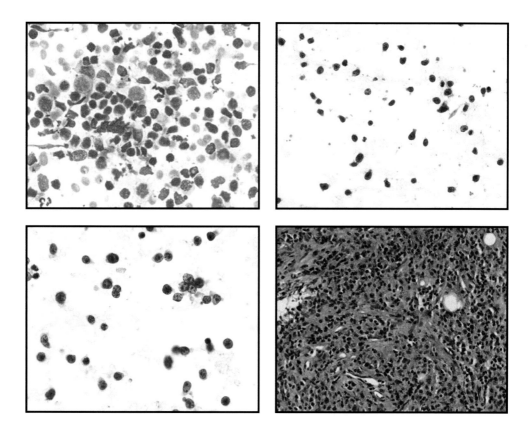

Clinical History

Fine needle aspiration biopsy of a kidney mass in a 75-year-old male who is status posttransplant.

Choose the Best Diagnosis

    a. Burkitt lymphoma

    b. Reactive lymphoid hyperplasia

    c. Renal cell carcinoma

    d. Posttransplant lymphoproliferative disorder (PTLD)

    e. Chronic rejection

ANSWER AND BRIEF DISCUSSION

d. Posttransplant Lymphoproliferative Disorder (PTLD)

The specimen reveals predominantly lymphoid cells. The lymphoid cells are enlarged but display a polymorphous pattern.

In the setting of a renal transplant, the presence of numerous lymphocytes in this transplanted kidney raises the possibility of a lymphoproliferative disorder. Although the lymphoid population is polymorphous, the presence of predominantly moderate to large cells suggests that this is not simply a reactive process. There are a large number of plasmacytoid cells present that can be seen in PTLD. Immunophenotyping failed to identify a clonal population. Ultimately, an open biopsy was performed of this lesion, which revealed a plasmacytoma-like monomorphous variant of PTLD. An immunostain for Epstein-Barr virus latent membrane protein was focally positive in the larger immunoblastic cells. In situ hybridization was diffusely positive.

References

1. Subhawong AP, Subhawong TK, VandenBussche CJ, Siddiqui MT, Ali SZ. Lymphoproliferative disorders of the kidney on fine-needle aspiration: cytomorphology and radiographic correlates in 33 cases. *Acta Cytol*. 2013;57(1):19–25.
2. Gattuso P, Castelli MJ, Peng Y, Reddy VB. Posttransplant lymphoproliferative disorders: a fine-needle aspiration biopsy study. *Diagn Cytopathol*. 1997;16(5):392–395.

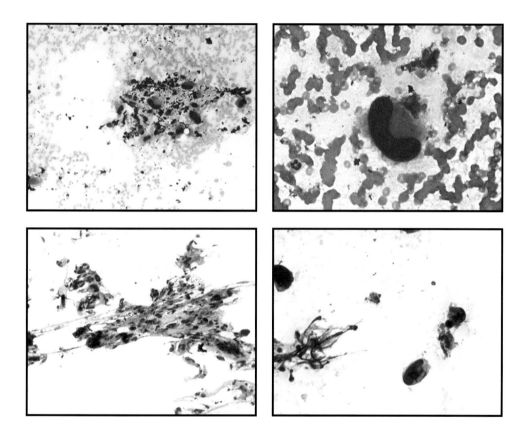

Clinical History

Fine needle aspiration (FNA) biopsy of a liver mass in a 17-year-old male.

Choose the Best Diagnosis

a. Metastatic osteosarcoma

b. Adenocarcinoma

c. Hepatoblastoma

d. Hepatocellular carcinoma (HCC)

e. Metastatic melanoma

ANSWER AND BRIEF DISCUSSION

a. Metastatic Osteosarcoma

This specimen contains scattered large atypical cells arranged singly and in small clusters. The cells have large pleomorphic nuclei with prominent nucleoli and delicate cytoplasm. In addition, there is focal acellular metachromatically staining matrix in the background.

The pleomorphic nature of these cells immediately suggests that this is a poorly differentiated malignant neoplasm. The cytoplasm gives some clues to the nature of these cells. The cells contain abundant delicate cytoplasm that has fine cytoplasmic projections radiating away from the nucleus. In addition, some of these cells are fusiform in shape with bipolar projections of cytoplasm. These features suggest a sarcomatous origin. In addition, there is focal acellular material in the background that suggests osteoid or perhaps chondroid matrix. Taken together, these findings are suggestive of a metastatic sarcoma such as osteosarcoma. Pleomorphic malignant cells in a liver FNA in a relatively young male should also raise the possibility of a fibrolamellar variant of HCC; however, this specimen is not entirely consistent with that entity.

References

1. Collins BT, Cramer HM, Ramos RR. Fine needle aspiration biopsy of recurrent and metastatic osteosarcoma. *Acta Cytol*. 1998;42(2):357–361.
2. Domanski HA, Akerman M. Fine-needle aspiration of primary osteosarcoma: a cytological-histological study. *Diagn Cytopathol*. 2005;32(5):269–275.

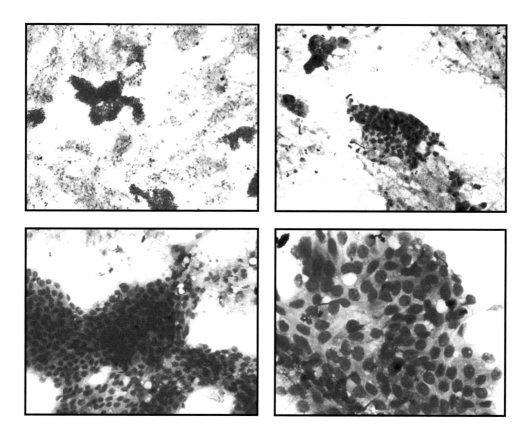

Clinical History

Fine needle aspiration of a liver lesion in a 76-year-old male with a history of infiltrating moderately differentiated adenocarcinoma of the colon and currently with a pancreatic mass and multiple lung nodules.

Choose the Best Diagnosis

a. Hepatocellular carcinoma

b. Metastatic adenocarcinoma, consistent with colonic primary

c. Metastatic carcinoma consistent with pancreatic primary

d. Poorly differentiated carcinoma

e. Metastatic neuroendocrine tumor

ANSWER AND BRIEF DISCUSSION

c. Metastatic Carcinoma Consistent With Pancreatic Primary

This specimen contains abundant necrosis as well as scattered atypical epithelial fragments that have glandular features. The nuclei within these fragments are large and pleomorphic.

There is an obvious metastatic adenocarcinoma in this liver. The major question concerns the site of origin in a patient with a history of colorectal carcinoma and a current pancreatic mass. Immunohistochemical stains can be very useful in sorting this out. In this case, the tumor was positive for CK7 and negative for CK20, DPC-4, and thyroid transcription factor-1. These findings argue against the metastasis from the patient's known colonic primary, which was floridly positive for both CK20 and CK7. Despite our reluctance to give patients a second primary, in this case, the immunohistochemical stains argue that this is indeed the case.

Reference

1. Cibas ES, Ducatman BS. *Cytology: Diagnostic Principles and Clinical Correlates.* 4th ed. Philadelphia, PA: Saunders; 2014:388–394.

CASE

50

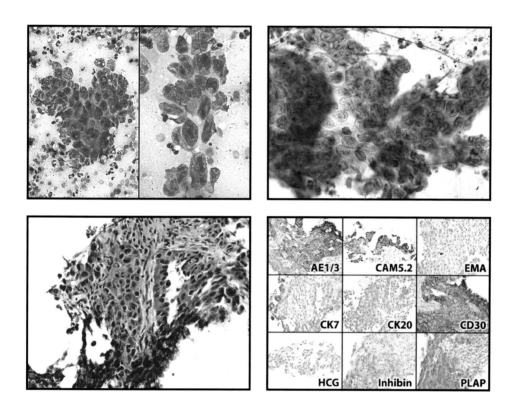

Clinical History

A 24-year-old man presents with dull abdominal pain that is unrelated to food intake. Physical exam shows enlargement of the right testis and an enlarged right supraclavicular lymph node. Abdominal CT reveals bulky lymphadenopathy of the periportal, periceliac, and aortic regions. Thoracic CT shows numerous areas of mediastinal and supraclavicular lymphadenopathy. Ultrasound-guided fine needle aspiration and core biopsy of right supraclavicular lymph node.

Choose the Best Diagnosis

a. Hodgkin lymphoma

b. Metastatic embryonal carcinoma

c. Thymoma

d. Rhabdomyosarcoma

e. Large cell lymphoma

ANSWER AND BRIEF DISCUSSION

b. Metastatic Embryonal Carcinoma

The aspirates show cohesive epithelial fragments having very large, markedly atypical cells with high N/C ratios, prominent single nucleoli, crowding, pleomorphism, and primitive glandular or acinar formations. There is no evidence of a mixed inflammatory cell background. Immunohistochemical stains are reactive for cytokeratin AE1/3, CAM 5.2, CK7, CD30, and PLAP. Immunostains are negative for CK20, EMA, HCG, and inhibin.

The clinical scenario of a young patient with multiple enlarged lymph nodes (in what may be a contiguous chain) gives a clinical suspicion of Hodgkin lymphoma, but the combination of immunoreactivity for both cytokeratin AE1/3 and CD30 makes embryonal carcinoma the most likely diagnosis.

Reference

1. Stanley MW, Powers CN, Pitman MB, Korourian S, Bardales RH, Khurana K. Cytology of germ cell tumors: extragonadal, extracranial masses and intraoperative problems. *Cancer.* 1997;81(4):220–227.

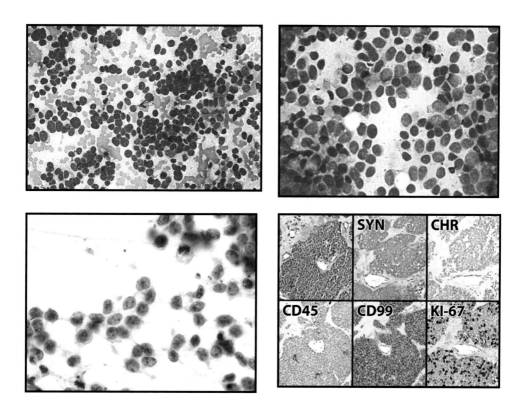

Clinical History

An 11-year-old boy presents with a swelling of the left lower leg. He reports that he was kicked in that area 4 months ago and has no residual pain or any other complaints. Physical exam reveals left calf fullness but no lymphadenopathy. Radiographs show a 7-cm soft-tissue mass emanating from an area of fibular destruction in the diaphysis. Ultrasound-guided fine needle aspiration and core biopsy of lower leg soft tissue mass.

Choose the Best Diagnosis

a. Ewing sarcoma/primitive neuroectodermal tumor (PNET)

b. Malignant lymphoma

c. Osteosarcoma

d. Rhabdomyosarcoma

e. Reactive lymph node

ANSWER AND BRIEF DISCUSSION

a. Ewing Sarcoma/Primitive Neuroectodermal Tumor (PNET)

The smears are cellular, and both single cells and large aggregates are present at low power. Some of these cells form rosette-like structures. At high power, the lesion comprises fairly monotonous, small round blue cells with scant cytoplasm, high N/C ratio, and multiple cytoplasmic vacuoles. The Papanicolaou-stained material demonstrates round to oval nuclei with multiple small nucleoli and occasional mitotic figures. Immunohistochemistry shows that the cells are immunoreactive for CD99 (O13/MIC2).

The differential diagnosis includes the small round blue cell tumors of childhood. Morphologically, small cell osteosarcomas can appear similar to Ewing sarcoma, but one would expect to find some osteoid formation. Other immunohistochemical stains that might have been helpful include desmin and myogenin (positive in rhabdomyosarcoma) and terminal deoxynucleotidyl transferase (TdT) (positive in lymphoblastic lymphoma). Also, cytogenetic studies in this case most likely would demonstrate a reciprocal translocation of chromosomes 11 and 22, leading to the production of the chimeric fusion gene EWS/FLI-1 in the majority of Ewing sarcoma cases. A minority of cases have translocations involving chromosome 22 (the locus of the EWS gene) with other ETS family transcription factor genes on chromosomes 21 (ERG), 7 (ETV1), 17 (ETV4), and 2 (FEV).

References

1. Lewis TB, Coffin CM, Bernard PS. Differentiating Ewing's sarcoma from other round blue cell tumors using a RT-PCR translocation panel on formalin-fixed paraffin-embedded tissues. *Mod Pathol*. 2007;20(3):397–404.
2. Renshaw AA, Perez-Atayde AR, Fletcher JA, Granter SR. Cytology of typical and atypical Ewing's sarcoma/PNET. *AJCP*. 1996;106(5):620–624.

CASE

52

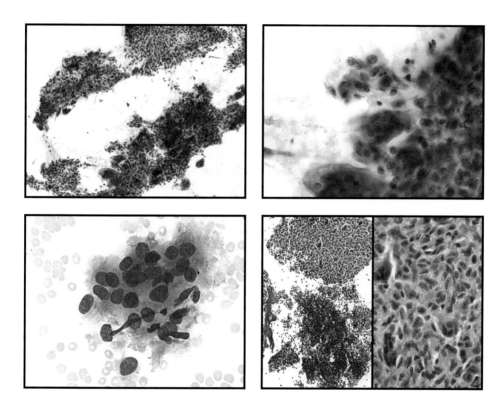

Clinical History

A 26-year-old woman presents with a 6-month history of an enlarging mass in the left calf. She denies any history of trauma. Plain radiographs show a lytic lesion in the epiphysis and metaphysis of the proximal fibula with extension into the calf, forming a large soft-tissue mass. Fine needle aspiration of a left proximal fibula mass with core needle biopsy.

Choose the Best Diagnosis

a. Granulomatous inflammation

b. Osteosarcoma

c. Giant cell tumor

d. Malignant fibrous histiocytoma

e. Melanoma

ANSWER AND BRIEF DISCUSSION

c. Giant Cell Tumor

The aspirate and core biopsy show numerous fairly uniform cells with abundant cytoplasm, occasional small cytoplasmic vacuoles, oval to round nuclei, and rare small nucleoli. Intermixed are numerous multinucleated giant cells showing similar nuclear and cytoplasmic features. No significant lymphocytic or neutrophilic infiltrate is identified. Mitotic activity is low, and no abnormal mitoses or frankly sarcomatous areas are identified.

The radiographic and microscopic features are most compatible with a giant cell tumor. The resemblance of the individual giant cell nuclei to the nuclei of the surrounding stromal cells is distinctive, while the overwhelming number of giant cells and lack of granuloma formation argues against granulomatous inflammation. Although giant cell tumors are locally aggressive, the benign histologic features here are insufficient for a diagnosis of malignancy. Surgical resection reveals a 12-cm giant cell tumor with aneurysmal bone cyst changes.

References

1. Sneige N, Ayala AG, Carrasco CH, Murray J, Raymond AK. Giant cell tumor of bone. A cytologic study of 24 cases. *Diagn Cytopathol.* 1985;1(2):111–117.
2. Vetrani A, Fulciniti F, Boschi R, et al. Fine needle aspiration biopsy diagnosis of giant-cell tumor of bone. An experience with nine cases. *Acta Cytol.* 1990;34(6):863–867.

CASE

53

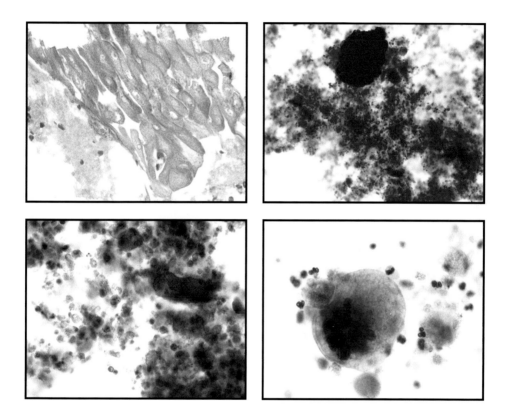

Clinical History

This cyst fluid is from a brain mass in a 41-year-old man. He presents to the emergency department with short-term memory loss and is found to have a cystic and partially solid mass extending from the suprasellar cistern into the third ventricle.

Choose the Best Diagnosis

    a. Rathke's cleft cyst

    b. Glioblastoma multiforme

    c. Pilocytic astrocytoma

    d. Craniopharyngioma

    e. Cysticercosis

ANSWER AND BRIEF DISCUSSION

d. Craniopharyngioma

The smears show anucleate "ghost cells," squamous debris, calcifications, and giant cells. No ciliated epithelium is identified.

Craniopharyngiomas are the most common suprasellar tumors in children and are derived from the embryonic nasopharynx (Rathke's pouch) that migrates to form the anterior part of the hypophysis. The differential includes epidermoid cyst (fibrous wall lined by keratinizing squamous epithelium; contains squames but no skin adnexa or hair) and Rathke's cleft cyst (respiratory epithelium with varying degrees of squamous metaplasia). There are two types of craniopharyngiomas: adamantinomatous (calcified, "motor oil" wet keratin, more frequent in children) and papillary (more common in adults and confers a better prognosis due to decreased frequency of recurrence). Although these lesions are benign, they are difficult to resect completely.

Reference

1. Parwani AV, Taylor DC, Burger PC, Erozan YS, Olivi A, Ali SZ. Keratinized squamous cells in fine needle aspiration of the brain. Cytopathologic correlates and differential diagnosis. *Acta Cytol.* 2003;47(3):325–331.

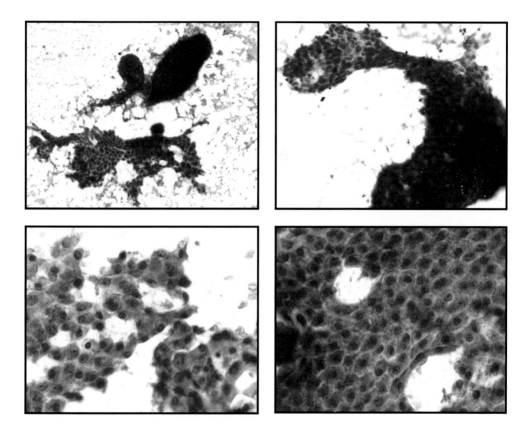

Clinical History

A 46-year-old female with biopsy-proven ductal carcinoma, lower outer quadrant. This is a fine needle aspiration from a second hypoechoic focus in the upper inner quadrant of the same breast.

Choose the Best Diagnosis

a. Ductal carcinoma, NOS

b. Apocrine carcinoma

c. Benign apocrine metaplasia

d. Metastatic malignant melanoma

e. Granular cell tumor

ANSWER AND BRIEF DISCUSSION

c. Benign Apocrine Metaplasia

Papanicolaou-stained slides show sheets of epithelial cells with granular and eosinophilic cytoplasm. These cells have sharply defined cytoplasmic borders. The nuclei are round and oval, and each has a single round nucleus. Their N/C ratios are low. No significant numbers of single epithelioid cells with cytoplasm are seen.

Despite the known history of ductal carcinoma in the same breast, the presence of abundant apocrine metaplasia is suggestive of a benign diagnosis. Breast carcinoma can rarely show apocrine phenotype, and there are no features of malignancy in this specimen. There is abundant cellularity, but given the patient's relatively young age, the significance of this is unclear. Occasional sheets show staghorn-like outlines. Others show more papillary features. While these findings may represent a fibroadenoma or intraductal papilloma, such a distinction is not important in this clinical scenario.

References

1. Stanley MW, Sidawy MK, Sanchez MA, Stahl RE, Goldfischer M. Current issues in breast cytopathology. *AJCP*. 2000;113(5 suppl 1):S49–S75.
2. Maygarden SJ, Novotny DB, Johnson DE, Frable WJ. Subclassification of benign breast disease by fine needle aspiration cytology. Comparison of cytologic and histologic findings in 265 palpable breast masses. *Acta Cytol*. 1994;38(2):115–129.

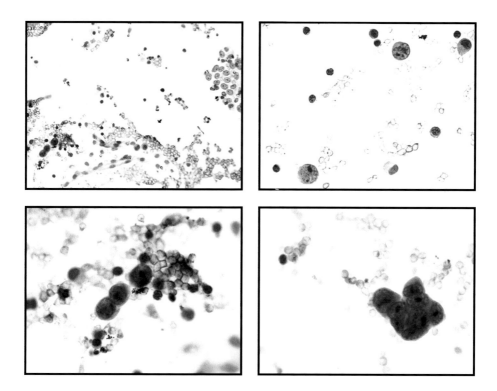

Clinical History

A 14-year-old girl presents with a 3- to 4-month history of increasing abdominal girth and abdominal pain. Laboratory workup showed the following: HCG 89 mIU/mL, CA-125 21 U/mL, AFP 2 ng/mL, and LDH 1071 U/L. Ultrasound demonstrates no intrauterine pregnancy, but does reveal a 17-cm left ovarian mass. During the left salpingo-oophorectomy, pelvic wash material is submitted for cytologic examination. Cytospin of intraoperative pelvic wash.

Choose the Best Diagnosis

a. Reactive mesothelial cells

b. Mesothelioma

c. Malignant neoplasm, favor dysgerminoma

d. Malignant neoplasm, favor embryonal carcinoma

e. Large cell lymphoma

ANSWER AND BRIEF DISCUSSION

c. Malignant Neoplasm, Favor Dysgerminoma

The pelvic wash shows a background of red blood cells with scattered lymphocytes and macrophages. Fragments and small sheets of benign reactive mesothelial cells also are present. However, within this background, there are several distinctive fragments and single cells that are large and round with high N/C ratios, scant cytoplasm, fine to slightly clumped chromatin, thick nuclear membranes, and prominent nucleoli.

This is a difficult case due to the scant amount of diagnostic material and the absence of helpful clues that one would see in a more abundant aspiration. For instance, the classic "tigroid" background of dysgerminomas/seminomas (seen on fine needle aspiration) is not present, nor is there the typical admixed lymphocytic population. However, compared to dysgerminomas, embryonal carcinomas tend to be more cohesive and show more pleomorphism. The presence of psammoma bodies and papillary architecture would have favored a diagnosis of serous carcinoma. Immunohistochemically, poorly differentiated carcinoma and embryonal carcinoma would be immunoreactive for cytokeratin, while dysgerminomas are nonreactive. The surgical resection revealed a 20-cm dysgerminoma of the left ovary.

References

1. Akhtar M, Ali MA, Huq M, Bakry M. Fine-needle aspiration biopsy of seminoma and dysgerminoma: cytologic, histologic, and electron microscopic correlations. *Diagn Cytopathol.* 1990;6(2):99–105.
2. Stanley MW, Powers CN, Pitman MB, Korourian S, Bardales RH, Khurana K. Cytology of germ cell tumors: extragonadal, extracranial masses and intraoperative problems. *Cancer.* 1997;81(4): 220–227.

CASE

56

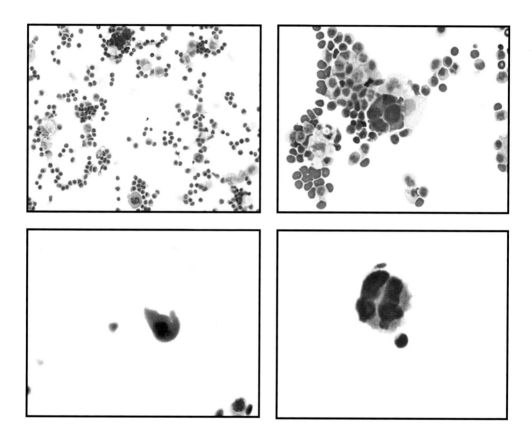

Clinical History

Cerebrospinal fluid (CSF) cytology from a 43-year-old female with a cancer history.

Choose the Best Diagnosis

    a. Hodgkin lymphoma

    b. High-grade astrocytoma

    c. Metastatic malignant melanoma

    d. Metastatic non-small cell carcinoma

    e. Peripheral T-cell lymphoma

ANSWER AND BRIEF DISCUSSION

d. Metastatic Non-Small Cell Carcinoma

Diff-Quik and Papanicolaou-stained slides show a cellular field with numerous lymphocytes, plasma cells, and red cells with scattered cellular clusters of atypical epithelioid cells. At scanning power, these clusters of cells are clearly malignant and occasional mitotic figures are identified. On the Pap-stained slide, occasional malignant cells show a somewhat "hard" cytoplasm suggestive of squamous differentiation.

Given the overall cellularity in this CSF, the primary distinction to be made is that between a hematopoietic and nonhematopoietic malignancy. In this case, the patient had a history of cervical squamous cell carcinoma, thus favoring a nonhematopoietic malignancy. Other features supporting that in this specimen are the close clustering of epithelioid malignant cells with hard cytoplasm. The epithelioid nature of the cells argues against a hematopoietic malignancy such as Hodgkin lymphoma or T-cell lymphoma involving the brain, which could otherwise account for the marked atypia. The close clustering of the malignant cells also argues against a primary brain tumor as well as a metastatic malignant melanoma.

Reference

1. Glantz MJ, Cole BF, Glantz LK, et al. Cerebrospinal fluid cytology in patients with cancer. *Cancer.* 1998;82(4):733–739.

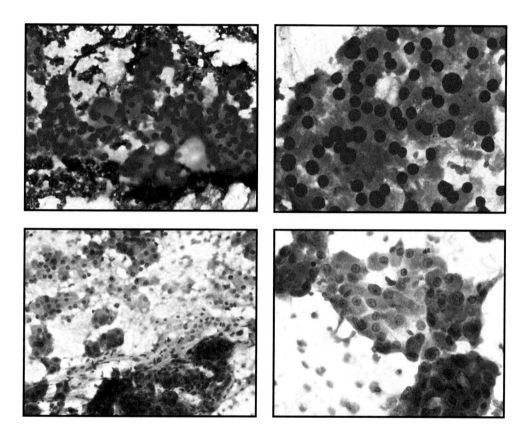

Clinical History

A 22-year-old female with thyroid nodule. Fine-needle aspiration.

Choose the Best Diagnosis

a. Hashimoto thyroiditis

b. Suspicious for a Hurthle cell neoplasm

c. Papillary thyroid carcinoma

d. Adenomatoid nodule

e. Medullary thyroid carcinoma

ANSWER AND BRIEF DISCUSSION

b. Suspicious for a Hurthle Cell Neoplasm

Diff-Quik and Papanicolaou-stained smears show loose sheets and discohesive spreads of granular cells with round nuclei. There is little to no background colloid, and overall, the cellularity is high. There are a few normal-appearing follicles. There is focal anisonucleosis but no features suggestive of papillary carcinoma (no nuclear inclusions, no grooves, and no significant nuclear overlap).

The features are that of a Hurthle cell neoplasm. While there are no overt features of malignancy, the biologic behavior of Hurthle cell neoplasms is unpredictable based on cytologic features alone. Hurthle cell features can be seen focally in other lesions such as adenomatoid nodules and Hashimoto thyroiditis. In this case, only Hurthle cells are seen throughout. Upon surgical resection, focal vascular invasion was seen, and the specimen was diagnosed as a minimally invasive Hurthle cell carcinoma.

Reference

1. Cibas ES, Ali SZ. The Bethesda system for reporting thyroid cytopathology. *Thyroid*. 2009;19(11): 1159–1165.

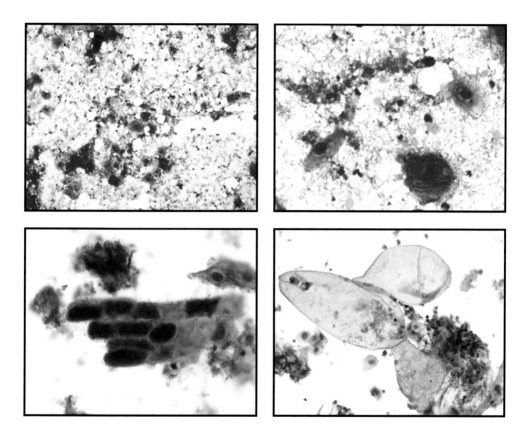

Clinical History

A 60-year-old female with left thyroid nodule. She has a history of a meningioma in the left sinus. Fine needle aspiration of the thyroid mass.

Choose the Best Diagnosis

a. Thyroglossal duct cyst

b. Squamous cell carcinoma

c. Branchial cleft cyst

d. Oropharyngeal diverticulum

e. Meningioma

ANSWER AND BRIEF DISCUSSION

d. Oropharyngeal Diverticulum

Diff-Quik and Papanicolaou-stained smears show scattered mature squamous cells, filamentous bacteria, fungal forms, and vegetable (food) material. No thyroid tissue is identified.

The presence of vegetable material and lack of respiratory epithelium are highly suggestive of an oropharyngeal diverticulum (Killian-Jamieson diverticulum). Killian-Jamieson and Zenker diverticula are outpouchings in the wall of the hypopharynx or cervical esophagus and may be in the vicinity of the thyroid gland. Rarely, these diverticula may present radiographically as a thyroid nodule. In addition to these diverticula, the differential diagnosis of oropharyngeal contents found at this site includes a thyroglossal duct fistula and pyriform sinus fistula.

Reference

1. Rekhtman N, Rekhtman K, Sheth S, Ali SZ. A 62-year-old woman with a suspected thyroid nodule: Killian-Jamieson diverticulum. *Arch Pathol Lab Med*. 2005;129(11):1497–1498.

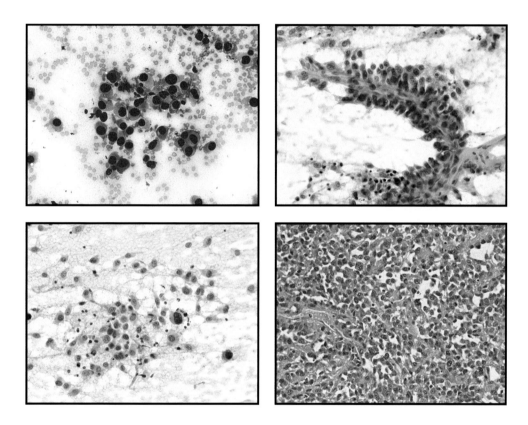

Clinical History

An 81-year-old male with parotid mass. Fine needle aspiration.

Choose the Best Diagnosis

    a. Pleomorphic adenoma

    b. Adenoid cystic carcinoma

    c. Warthin tumor

    d. Myoepithelioma

    e. Mucoepidermoid carcinoma

ANSWER AND BRIEF DISCUSSION

d. Myoepithelioma

Smears display loosely cohesive and dispersed epithelioid cells with slight pleomorphism. The cytoplasm is abundant, and in some instances, the cells have a plasmacytoid appearance. Nuclei are bland, ovoid, and without atypia or obvious nucleoli. No myxoid or chondroid material is seen in the background.

These features are consistent with a myoepithelioma, which was confirmed on excision of the tail of the parotid. The differential diagnosis in this case includes other monomorphic adenomas such as a basal cell adenoma and even a carotid body tumor in the appropriate radiographic setting. Basal cell adenomas may secrete a metachromatic hyaline-like material, which is not seen in this case. Myoepithelial cells are usually a component of major salivary gland tumors, and pure myoepitheliomas are rare, accounting for less than 1% of salivary gland neoplasms. Although usually pursuing a benign course, malignant myoepitheliomas have been described.

References

1. Dodd LG, Caraway NP, Luna MA, Byers RM. Myoepithelioma of the parotid. Report of a case initially examined by fine needle aspiration biopsy. *Acta Cytol.* 1994;38(3):417–421.
2. Stewart CJ, MacKenzie K, McGarry GW, Mowat A. Fine-needle aspiration cytology of salivary gland: a review of 341 cases. *Diagn Cytopathol.* 2000;22(3):139–146.

CASE

60

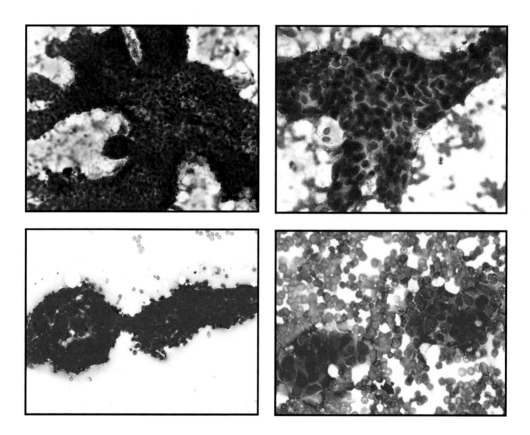

Clinical History

A 36-year-old woman with a palpable, mobile breast mass. Fine needle aspiration.

Choose the Best Diagnosis

    a. Ductal carcinoma

    b. Fibroadenoma

    c. Lactational change

    d. Metastatic melanoma

    e. Adenomyoepithelioma

ANSWER AND BRIEF DISCUSSION

b. Fibroadenoma

The smears display a moderate- to high-cellularity specimen with numerous branching fingerlike fragments. No foam cells or apocrine changes are identified. Some clusters of ductal epithelium surrounded by naked nuclei are identified; no frank atypia is noted.

The cytomorphologic features are quite characteristic for a fibroadenoma (sheets of cohesive epithelial cells, branching antler horn fragments, a few bipolar naked nuclei, and stromal fragments). Even when aspiration of a breast mass produces a hypercellular specimen, a diagnosis of malignancy should not be made unless multiple cytologic criteria are present.

References

1. Benoit JL, Kara R, McGregor SE, Duggan MA. Fibroadenoma of the breast: diagnostic pitfalls of fine-needle aspiration. *Diagn Cytopathol.* 1992;8(6):643–647.
2. Maygarden SJ, Novotny DB, Johnson DE, Frable WJ. Subclassification of benign breast disease by fine needle aspiration cytology. Comparison of cytologic and histologic findings in 265 palpable breast masses. *Acta Cytol.* 1994;38(2):115–129.

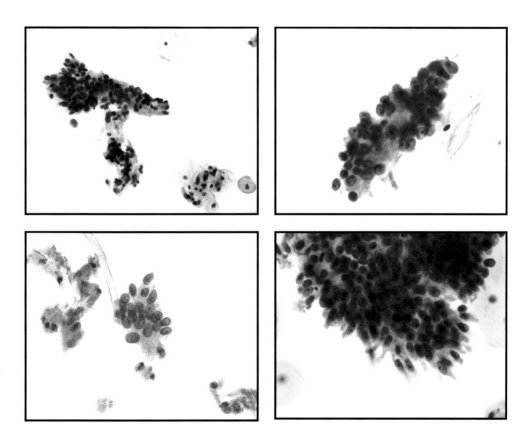

Clinical History

Liquid-based Papanicolaou test (SurePath) in a 56-year-old woman.

Choose the Best Diagnosis

    a. Adenocarcinoma in-situ (AIS)

    b. Atypical glandular cells

    c. Atypical squamous cells of undetermined significance

    d. Endometrial adenocarcinoma

    e. Reactive cellular changes

ANSWER AND BRIEF DISCUSSION

a. Adenocarcinoma In-Situ (AIS)

Numerous hyperchromatic, crowded groups of glandular cells with feathered edges are present. The glandular cells appear markedly atypical with enlarged nuclei, increased N/C ratios, and coarse chromatin. Some of the cells have discernible nucleoli. The background is relatively clean.

The described changes are beyond the realm of reactive and warrant a diagnosis of AIS. Endometrial lesions should be considered in this case, but the feathering of the edges of the fragments and clear polarization of some of the cells is more consistent with endocervical origin. Prominent nucleoli, which can be seen in invasive endocervical adenocarcinoma, can occasionally be noted in AIS, particularly in liquid-based preparations.

References

1. Sherman ME, Dasgupta A, Schiffman M, Nayar R, Solomon D. The Bethesda Interobserver Reproducibility Study (BIRST): a web-based assessment of the Bethesda 2001 System for classifying cervical cytology. *Cancer.* 2007;111(1):15–25.
2. Solomon D, Nayar R. *The Bethesda System for Reporting Cervical Cytology: Definitions, Criteria, and Explanatory Notes.* 2nd ed. New York, NY: Springer; 2006:123–156.

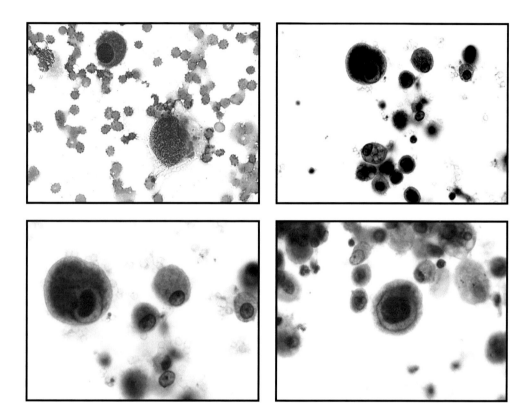

Clinical History

A 50-year-old woman with a history of acute myeloid leukemia presents with a 2-day history of upper respiratory tract symptoms, fever, and productive cough. CT of the chest reveals bilateral diffuse micronodular and "ground glass" infiltrates. Bronchoalveolar lavage.

Choose the Best Diagnosis

    a. Acute myeloid leukemia

    b. Cytomegalovirus infection

    c. Ehrlichiosis

    d. Leishmaniasis

    e. Histoplasmosis

ANSWER AND BRIEF DISCUSSION

b. Cytomegalovirus Infection

The smears show mainly red blood cells in the background with scattered mononuclear cells. There is a subpopulation of cells having marked overall cellular enlargement, intracytoplasmic inclusions, and intranuclear inclusions with a surrounding halo. The nuclei in these cells are 3 to 4 times the size of nuclei in neighboring pulmonary alveolar macrophages. These features are consistent with CMV infection.

Leishmaniasis, ehrlichiosis, and histoplasmosis can have numerous small organisms in the cytoplasm of infected cells, but do not have intranuclear inclusions. In ehrlichiosis, these cytoplasmic inclusions often form a "morula" of organisms bound to a vacuole. While acute myeloid leukemia can have prominent nucleoli and Auer rods, the morphology of the inclusions shown is not compatible with leukemia.

Reference

1. Linder J, Vaughan WP, Armitage JO, et al. Cytopathology of opportunistic infection in bronchoalveolar lavage. *AJCP*. 1987;88(4):421–428.

CASE
63

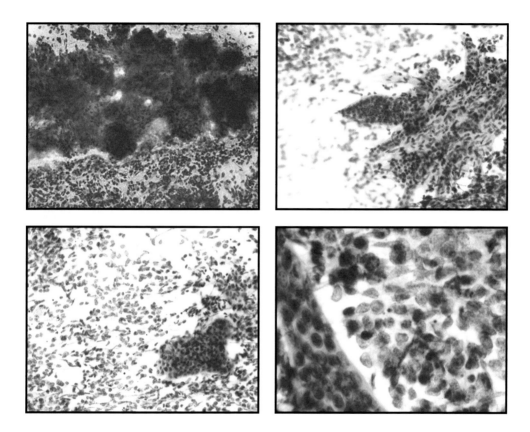

Clinical History

Fine needle aspiration of a kidney mass in a 2-year-old boy.

Choose the Best Diagnosis

a. Ossifying renal tumor of infancy

b. Clear cell sarcoma of kidney

c. Mesoblastic nephroma

d. Nephroblastoma

e. Benign renal tissue

ANSWER AND BRIEF DISCUSSION

d. Nephroblastoma

The aspirates are cellular and show a multiphasic tumor. Cohesive epithelial structures including nests and tubular structures predominate. Additionally, there are less cohesive blastemic cells adjacent to the epithelial cells with higher N/C ratios. Close inspection of the cohesive cellular fragments shows spindled mesenchymal cells between the nested epithelial elements.

This case is an excellent example of nephroblastoma (Wilms' tumor). Although the other tumors listed as answer choices are pediatric renal tumors, only Wilms' tumor would show triphasic morphology. In addition to cytomorphologic differences, there are useful discriminating clinical features of the pediatric renal tumors. Nephroblastoma (Wilms' tumor) is the most common pediatric renal tumor. It is usually diagnosed between ages 2 and 5 and is uncommon in infants less than 6 months old. The pattern of metastases is often predictable, with spread to the regional lymph nodes, liver, and lung. Involvement of bone is unusual and should lead one to question the diagnosis of Wilms' tumor.

Mesoblastic nephroma is a congenital neoplasm and is the most common renal tumor in infants less than 6 months old. It has the same genetic translocation t(12;15) (p13;q25) that results in ETV6-NTRK3 gene fusion that is seen in infantile fibrosarcoma. Nephrectomy is usually curative. Clear cell sarcoma of kidney has its highest incidence in the second year of life. It commonly spreads to bone and has been called bone metastasizing renal tumor of childhood. Despite its name, clear cytoplasm is not a frequent finding. Ossifying renal tumor of infancy is an extremely rare tumor that is notable for calcification and osteoid matrix.

References

1. Radhika S, Bakshi A, Rajwanshi A, et al. Cytopathology of uncommon malignant renal neoplasms in the pediatric age group. *Diagn Cytopathol*. 2005;32(5):281–286.
2. Portugal R, Barroca H. Clear cell sarcoma, cellular mesoblastic nephroma and metanephric adenoma: cytological features and differential diagnosis with Wilms tumour. *Cytopathology*. 2008;19(2):80–85.

CASE

64

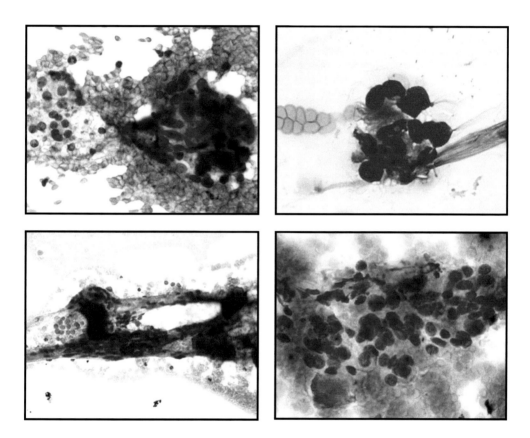

Clinical History

Thyroid fine needle aspiration in a 64-year-old female with a thyroid nodule.

Choose the Best Diagnosis

    a. Adenomatoid nodule

    b. Suspicious for a follicular neoplasm

    c. Suspicious for a Hurthle cell neoplasm

    d. Suspicious for papillary thyroid carcinoma (PTC)

    e. Hyalinizing trabecular neoplasm

ANSWER AND BRIEF DISCUSSION

d. Suspicious for Papillary Thyroid Carcinoma (PTC)

Diff-Quik and Papanicolaou-stained smears show a cellular aspirate with minimal colloid. A few small groups of normal follicular cells are seen. The majority of the cells are markedly enlarged, elongated, and overlapping. No nuclear grooves or inclusions are seen. The chromatin of this atypical population is powdery with one to two chromocenters. Small clumps of "hard" colloid are seen admixed with this cell population in areas.

Although the "classic" cytologic findings of PTC are not seen in this aspirate (nuclear grooves, intranuclear inclusions, and papillary structures), the oblong nuclear shape, nuclear overlapping, and powdery chromatin are highly suggestive of that diagnosis. The surgical resection showed multiple foci of PTC, follicular variant. As in the cytopathologic material, the nuclear features in the surgical resection displayed powdery chromatin with distinct chromocenters, but does not show grooves and inclusions.

Reference

1. Baloch ZW, LiVolsi VA, Asa SL, et al. Diagnostic terminology and morphologic criteria for cytologic diagnosis of thyroid lesions: a synopsis of the National Cancer Institute thyroid fine-needle aspiration state of the science conference. *Diagn Cytopathol.* 2008;36(6):425–437.

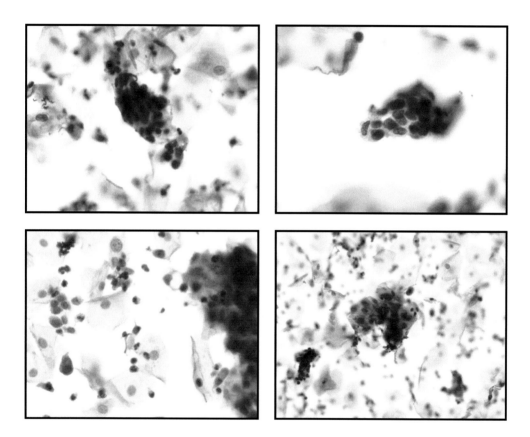

Clinical History

Liquid-based Papanicolaou test (SurePath) on a 52-year-old female with a history of high-grade squamous intraepithelial lesion (HSIL).

Choose the Best Diagnosis

a. Atypical glandular cells

b. Atypical squamous cells of undetermined significance (ASC-US)

c. HSIL

d. Low-grade squamous intraepithelial lession

e. Negative for intraepithelial lesion and malignancy

ANSWER AND BRIEF DISCUSSION

b. Atypical Squamous Cells of Undetermined Significance (ASC-US)

There is some parabasal atrophy. There are numerous fragments and individual cells that appear atypical. Many of the fragments are thick and obscure, though there is a suggestion of hyperchromasia and nuclear contour irregularities. Some individual squamous cells have markedly enlarged though somewhat degenerated nuclei. Many fragments show overtly reactive changes.

The best cytologic interpretation is ASC-US. Given the lack of koilocytes, lack of overtly high-grade features, and the significant reactive changes, a more definitive diagnosis is not rendered. Given this patient's history of HSIL, she was directly referred to colposcopy. Follow-up biopsy showed an extensive high-grade squamous epithelial lesion.

Reference

1. Sherman ME, Dasgupta A, Schiffman M, Nayar R, Solomon D. The Bethesda Interobserver Reproducibility Study (BIRST): a web-based assessment of the Bethesda 2001 System for classifying cervical cytology. *Cancer.* 2007;111(1):15–25.

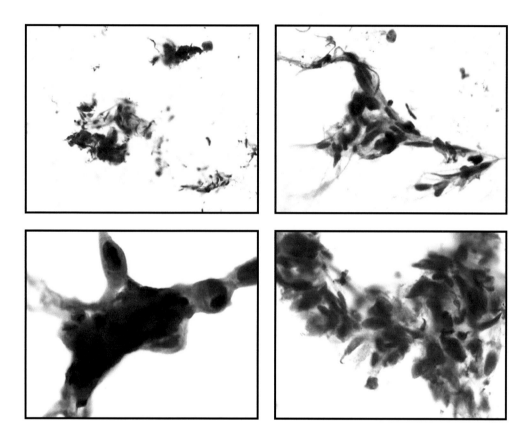

Clinical History

A 59-year-old female with abnormal bimanual exam. SurePath Papanicolaou (Pap) test.

Choose the Best Diagnosis

a. Invasive cervical adenocarcinoma

b. High-grade squamous intraepithelial lesion

c. Squamous cell carcinoma

d. Reactive epithelial changes

e. Atypical squamous cells of undetermined significance

ANSWER AND BRIEF DISCUSSION

c. Squamous Cell Carcinoma

The Pap slide is satisfactory for evaluation. Fragments of hyperchromatic crowded groups are present as well as single atypical cells with high N/C ratios. A tumor diathesis is present, evident by the granular background of blood, fibrin, and necrotic debris. A few spindled orangeophilic cells are seen with enlarged, hyperchromatic nuclei.

Even from a very low power, this is a concerning specimen because of the abundant altered blood in the background, suggestive of a tumor diathesis. The markedly atypical keratinizing cells are highly suspicious for squamous cell carcinoma. The necrosis and altered blood raise the possibility of invasion, which was present on subsequent cervical biopsy.

References

1. Sherman ME, Dasgupta A, Schiffman M, Nayar R, Solomon D. The Bethesda Interobserver Reproducibility Study (BIRST): a web-based assessment of the Bethesda 2001 System for classifying cervical cytology. *Cancer.* 2007;111(1):15–25.
2. Solomon D, Nayar R. *The Bethesda System for Reporting Cervical Cytology: Definitions, Criteria, and Explanatory Notes.* 2nd ed. New York, NY: Springer; 2006:89–122.

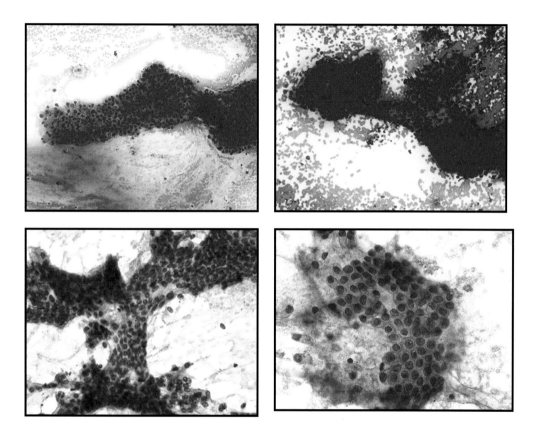

Clinical History

A 75-year-old female with recurrent pancreatitis and abnormal endoscopic retrograde cholangiopancreatography. Fine needle aspiration (FNA) of the pancreas.

Choose the Best Diagnosis

a. Adenocarcinoma arising in an intraductal papillary mucinous neoplasm (IPMN)

b. Benign ductal epithelium

c. Solid pseudopapillary neoplasm (SPN)

d. Metastatic ovarian serous carcinoma

e. Acinar cell carcinoma

ANSWER AND BRIEF DISCUSSION

a. Adenocarcinoma Arising in an IPMN

FNA displays cohesive epithelial sheets with papillary-like architecture. Nuclear enlargement and pleomorphism is evident. The background is composed predominantly of red cells and mucin.

This is clearly an adenocarcinoma of the pancreas, and the cytomorphologic features suggest that it arose in an IPMN. The differential diagnosis of such a lesion includes a mucinous cystic neoplasm, a pancreatic pseudocyst, and an SPN. The peak incidence for IPMN is in the sixth decade with a slight male predominance. They arise in the main pancreatic duct or one of its branches, and imaging studies assist in identifying their location.

References

1. Pitman MB. Revised international consensus guidelines for the management of patients with mucinous cysts. *Cancer Cytopathol*. 2012;120(6):361–365.
2. Stelow EB, Stanley MW, Bardales RH, et al. Intraductal papillary-mucinous neoplasm of the pancreas. The findings and limitations of cytologic samples obtained by endoscopic ultrasound-guided fine-needle aspiration. *AJCP*. 2003;120(3):398–404.

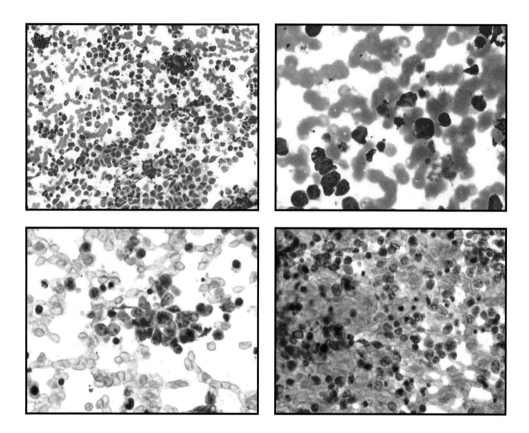

Clinical History

A 64-year-old female with mediastinal lymphadenopathy. Fine needle aspiration.

Choose the Best Diagnosis

a. Follicular lymphoma

b. Small cell carcinoma

c. Small lymphocytic lymphoma

d. Mantle cell lymphoma

e. Lymphoid hyperplasia

ANSWER AND BRIEF DISCUSSION

b. Small Cell Carcinoma

The aspirate is cellular with background lymphocytes and red blood cells. There is a loosely cohesive atypical small cell population with very high N/C ratios, finely granular "salt-and-pepper" chromatin, occasional mitoses, and apoptotic bodies. Occasionally, lymphoglandular bodies are seen in the background. There is prominent nuclear molding seen both in Diff-Quik and Papanicolaou-stained smears.

Reference

1. Travis WD, Rush W, Flieder DB, et al. Survival analysis of 200 pulmonary neuroendocrine tumors with clarification of criteria for atypical carcinoid and its separation from typical carcinoid. *Am J Surg Pathol.* 1998;22(8):934–944.

CASE

69

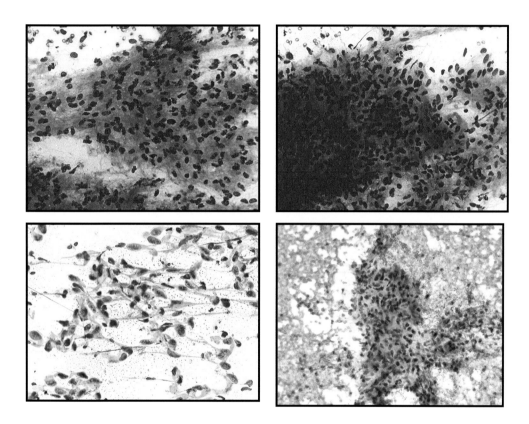

Clinical History

A 32-year-old with history of neurofibromatosis and shortness of breath. Fine needle aspiration of an inguinal mass. An S-100 protein immunostain is provided.

Choose the Best Diagnosis

a. Granulomatous inflammation

b. Metastatic adenocarcinoma

c. Malignant peripheral nerve sheath tumor (MPNST)

d. Malignant melanoma

e. Langerhans cell histiocytosis

ANSWER AND BRIEF DISCUSSION

c. Malignant Peripheral Nerve Sheath Tumor (MPNST)

The aspirate is hypercellular and displays oval to plump spindly cells embedded in a loose metachromatic stromal matrix. Anisonucleosis is evident. Cytoplasmic borders are hardly discernable. No intracytoplasmic pigment, intranuclear inclusions or glandular architecture is evident. Lack of lymphoid background suggests that this is likely not an involvement of a lymph node.

As is usually the case, history provides a useful diagnostic adjunct. In this case, the patient has a history of multiple neurofibromas, the most recent being a posterofemoral nerve mass that is an MPNST. The patient was lost to follow-up, never received adjuvant therapy, and developed diffuse pulmonary metastasis and this malignant effusion. The positivity for S-100 protein in this case was helpful, as it tends to be negative in nearly 50% of cases of MPNST. They most commonly occur in the neck, extremities, buttock, retroperitoneum, and mediastinum (posterior). They are almost always deep-seated, only rarely arising from superficial neurofibromas, rarely reported in other organs, and 50% are associated with neurofibromatosis type 1 (von Recklinghausen's disease).

References

1. Klijanienko J, Caillaud JM, Lagace R, Vielh P. Cytohistologic correlations of 24 malignant peripheral nerve sheath tumor (MPNST) in 17 patients: the Institut Curie experience. *Diagn Cytopathol.* 2002;27(2):103–108.
2. Jimenez-Heffernan JA, Lopez-Ferrer P, Vicandi B, Hardisson D, Gamallo C, Viguer JM. Cytologic features of malignant peripheral nerve sheath tumor. *Acta Cytol.* 1999;43(2):175–183.

CASE

70

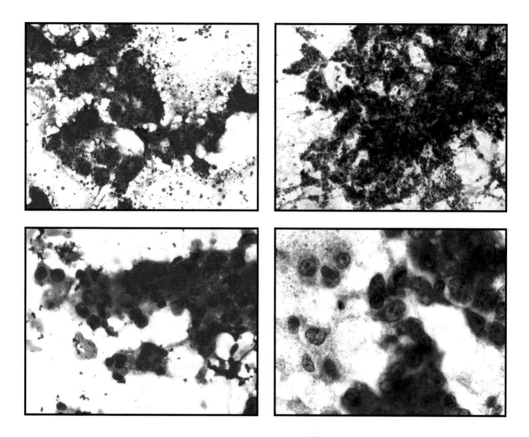

Clinical History

A 59-year-old with hepatitis C. Ultrasound-guided fine needle aspiration of a 4-cm liver mass.

Choose the Best Diagnosis

a. Hepatocellular carcinoma (HCC)

b. Hepatic adenoma

c. Metastatic adenocarcinoma consistent with pancreatic primary

d. Bile duct hamartoma

e. Benign hepatocytes with reactive changes

ANSWER AND BRIEF DISCUSSION

a. Hepatocellular Carcinoma (HCC)

Fine needle aspiration reveals thick plates and clusters of cells, some surrounding a fibrotic strand. These cells appear to be trabecular aggregates of hepatocytes, with dense granular cytoplasm and enlarged pleomorphic nuclei with prominent nucleoli. Examination of the specimen did not reveal bile duct epithelium.

HCC is reported to arise in 1 patient in 10 with cirrhosis (usually macronodular). HCC can be distinguished from adenomas in that HCC arises in a background of cirrhosis, whereas adenomas do not. Most patients with HCC are men (4:1) older than 60. Metastasis occurs in roughly 2/3 of cases, and HCC has a tendency to grow into vessels, even reaching the heart.

References

1. Wee A. Fine needle aspiration biopsy of the liver: algorithmic approach and current issues in the diagnosis of hepatocellular carcinoma. *CytoJournal*. 2005;2:7.
2. Takenaka A, Kaji I, Kasugai H, et al. Usefulness of diagnostic criteria for aspiration cytology of hepatocellular carcinoma. *Acta Cytol*. 1999;43(4):610–616.

CASE

71

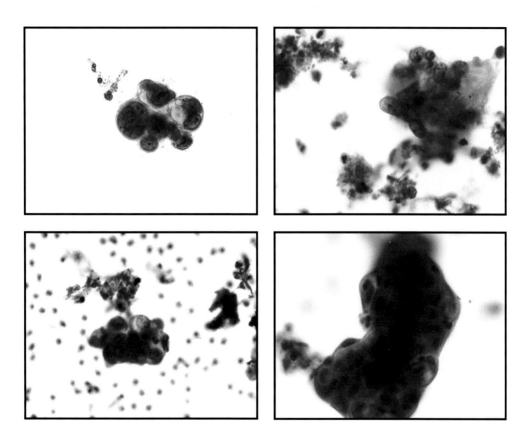

Clinical History

A 64-year-old female, status post total abdominal hysterectomy. Vaginal pool liquid-based Pap test (SurePath).

Choose the Best Diagnosis

a. Reactive changes secondary to intrauterine device

b. Adenocarcinoma

c. Atypical glandular cells

d. High-grade squamous intraepithelial lesion involving glands

e. Granulomatous inflammation

ANSWER AND BRIEF DISCUSSION

b. Adenocarcinoma

The cells are partially obscured by inflammation. The three-dimensionality of the fragments is difficult to appreciate on a static image. These aggregates are composed of atypical epithelial cells with hyperchromatic nuclei with irregular nuclear membranes. In one of the fragments, there is a cell harboring a mucin droplet, suggesting glandular differentiation.

Even though this smear exhibits scant cellularity and is partially obscured by inflammation, the presence of glandular cells in a vaginal pool specimen warrants concern. This patient had previously undergone resection of an endometrioid carcinoma that exhibited prominent mucinous differentiation.

References

1. Sherman ME, Dasgupta A, Schiffman M, Nayar R, Solomon D. The Bethesda Interobserver Reproducibility Study (BIRST): a web-based assessment of the Bethesda 2001 System for classifying cervical cytology. *Cancer.* 2007;111(1):15–25.
2. Solomon D, Nayar R. *The Bethesda System for Reporting Cervical Cytology: Definitions, Criteria, and Explanatory Notes.* 2nd ed. New York, NY: Springer; 2006:123–156.

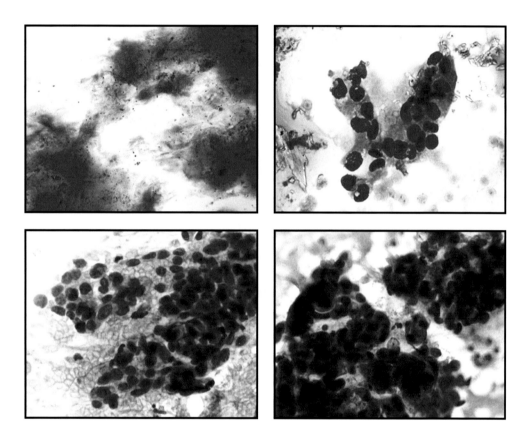

Clinical History

Pancreatic neck mass in a 52-year-old female. Endoscopic ultrasound-fine needle aspiration.

Choose the Best Diagnosis

a. Adenocarcinoma with mucinous features

b. Retention cyst with reactive ductal epithelial changes

c. Gastric contamination

d. Pseudocyst

e. Pancreatic neuroendocrine tumor

ANSWER AND BRIEF DISCUSSION

a. Adenocarcinoma With Mucinous Features

Aspirate smears show abundant mucin with scattered fragments of epithelial cells. These epithelial fragments are decidedly abnormal without the typical honeycomb pattern and regularity of normal ductal epithelium. There is significant anisonucleosis, three-dimensionality, and cellular atypia. On Papanicolaou stains, the nuclear chromatin is clumped and irregular.

These findings are consistent with a pancreatic mucinous neoplasm. These features could be seen in both an intraductal papillary mucinous neoplasm with high-grade dysplasia or underlying adenocarcinoma as well as in colloid carcinoma. On surgical follow-up, a moderate to poorly differentiated adenocarcinoma with prominent extracellular mucin and signet ring cells was resected.

References

1. Stelow EB, Stanley MW, Bardales RH, et al. Intraductal papillary-mucinous neoplasm of the pancreas. The findings and limitations of cytologic samples obtained by endoscopic ultrasound-guided fine-needle aspiration. *AJCP*. 2003;120(3):398–404.
2. Pitman MB. Revised international consensus guidelines for the management of patients with mucinous cysts. *Cancer Cytopathol*. 2012;120(6):361–365.

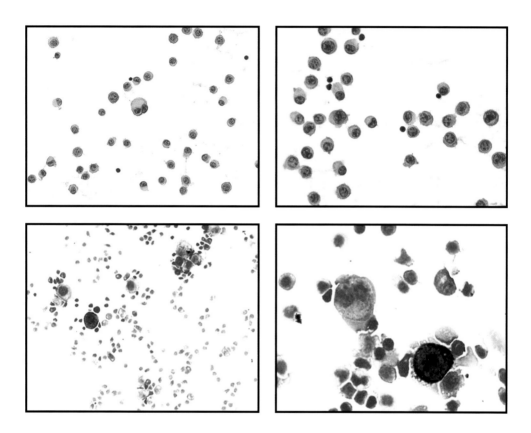

Clinical History

A 19-year-old male with ataxia and back pain. Cerebrospinal fluid (CSF).

Choose the Best Diagnosis

a. Glioblastoma multiforme

b. Metastatic melanoma

c. Primary central nervous system lymphoma

d. Changes consistent with cerebral infarct

e. Mollaret meningitis

ANSWER AND BRIEF DISCUSSION

b. Metastatic Melanoma

This CSF is markedly hypercellular. There are frequent large atypical cells with enlarged nuclei, and occasional double "mirror image" nucleated cells are seen. The cytoplasm of some of these cells contains pigment, suggestive of melanin. The background consists mainly of lymphocytes.

The primary melanoma in this 19-year-old was never discovered. Frequently, an ophthalmologic exam will reveal a retinal melanoma in such individuals, but occasionally the source of malignancy is a regressed cutaneous melanoma.

Reference

1. Prayson RA, Fischler DF. Cerebrospinal fluid cytology: an 11-year experience with 5951 specimens. *Arch Pathol Lab Med.* 1998;122(1):47–51.

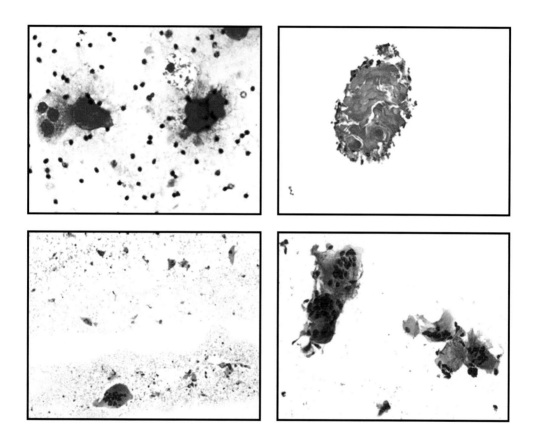

Clinical History

A 70-year-old male with diabetes insipidus and cystic suprasellar lesion. Fine needle aspiration of the brain mass.

Choose the Best Diagnosis

a. Craniopharyngioma

b. Metastatic squamous cell carcinoma

c. Neurosarcoidosis

d. Rathke's cleft cyst

e. Pinealoblastoma

ANSWER AND BRIEF DISCUSSION

a. Craniopharyngioma

Smears of the cyst contents display macrophages, occasional anucleate squames, granular debris, and multinucleated giant cells. A cytospin preparation of the fluid revealed a clump of "wet keratin" surrounded by squamous cells.

Derived from the embryonic craniopharyngeal canal (Rathke's pouch), craniopharyngiomas are the most common suprasellar tumors in children. The differential diagnosis in this case is an epidermoid cyst or a Rathke's cleft cyst, which contains respiratory epithelium with varying degrees of squamous metaplasia. Two types of craniopharyngiomas exist: adamantinomatous (calcified, "motor oil" wet keratin, more frequent in children) and papillary (more common in adults and confers a better prognosis due to decreased frequency of recurrence).

Reference

1. Parwani AV, Taylor DC, Burger PC, Erozan YS, Olivi A, Ali SZ. Keratinized squamous cells in fine needle aspiration of the brain. Cytopathologic correlates and differential diagnosis. *Acta Cytol.* 2003;47(3):325–331.

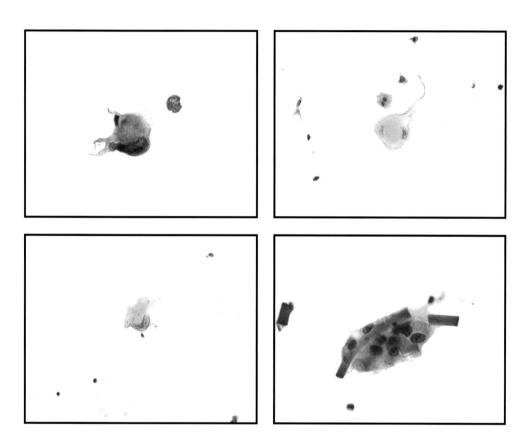

A 51-year-old patient, status post-hysterectomy 6 months ago. Vaginal pool liquid-based preparation (SurePath).

a. Atypical glandular cells, favor reactive changes secondary to intrauterine device

b. Carcinosarcoma

c. Radiation effect and suture granuloma

d. Low-grade squamous intraepithelial lesion

e. Squamous cell carcinoma

ANSWER AND BRIEF DISCUSSION

c. Radiation Effect and Suture Granuloma

Scattered throughout this vaginal pool specimen are markedly atypical cells with enlarged, irregular nuclei, but a preserved N/C ratio. Further inspection revealed foreign body giant cells surrounding suture material.

The history provides an important diagnostic clue in the evaluation of this specimen. Although there are wildly atypical cells present, the preservation of the N/C ratio raises our threshold for malignancy. It is important to note that the radiation effect may persist for life.

References

1. Bardales RH, Valente PT, Stanley MW. Cytology of suture granulomas in post-hysterectomy vaginal smears. *Diagn Cytopathol*. 1995;13(4):336–338.
2. Sherman ME, Dasgupta A, Schiffman M, Nayar R, Solomon D. The Bethesda Interobserver Reproducibility Study (BIRST): a web-based assessment of the Bethesda 2001 System for classifying cervical cytology. *Cancer*. 2007;111(1):15–25.

CASE
76

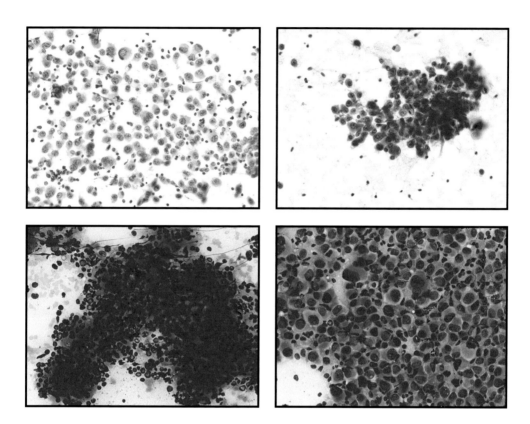

Fine needle aspiration of retroperitoneal mass in a 37-year-old female.

Choose the Best Diagnosis

a. Clear cell renal cell carcinoma

b. Metastatic melanoma

c. Leiomyosarcoma

d. Epithelioid angiomyolipoma

e. Teratoma

ANSWER AND BRIEF DISCUSSION

d. Epithelioid Angiomyolipoma

The specimen consists of sheets of quite atypical cells with enlarged, pleomorphic nuclei, course irregular chromatin, prominent nucleoli, and abundant eosinophilic granular cytoplasm, which was best seen in the cell block section. These findings are concerning for malignancy, and the differential in this case would include such entities as leiomyosarcoma, liposarcoma, and sarcomatoid renal cell carcinoma.

Although the cytologic findings are concerning, a positive immunohistochemical staining for HMB-45, in this case suggested an angiomyolipoma. This benign neoplasm, aptly named based on morphology, typically is composed of benign elements that befit its name in varying proportions. However, the recently recognized epithelioid variant has bizarre, large polygonal to short spindle cells that may be confused with sarcomas or carcinomas. Positive immunostaining for HMB-45 and the absence of epithelial markers is extremely helpful in the epithelial variant.

References

1. Zardawi IM. Renal fine needle aspiration cytology. *Acta Cytol.* 1999;43(2):184–190.
2. Mojica WD, Jovanoska S, Bernacki EG. Epithelioid angiomyolipoma: appearance on fine-needle aspiration report of a case. *Diagn Cytopathol.* 2000;23(3):192–195.

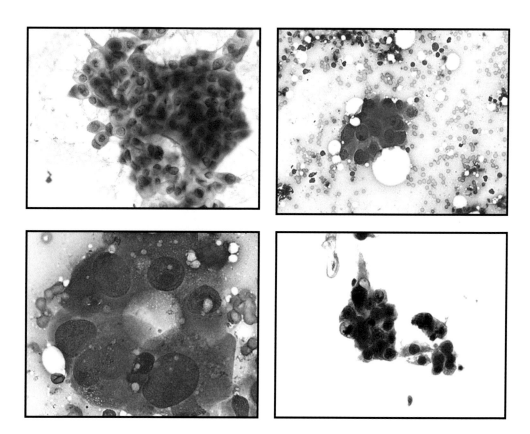

Clinical History

Fine needle aspiration of parotid lesion in a 65-year-old male.

Choose the Best Diagnosis

a. Pleomorphic adenoma

b. Salivary duct carcinoma

c. Chronic sialadenitis with reactive atypia

d. Adenoid cystic carcinoma

e. Squamous cell carcinoma

ANSWER AND BRIEF DISCUSSION

b. Salivary Duct Carcinoma

This cellular specimen is notable for sheets of epithelial cells with large round nuclei, prominent nucleoli, and abundant granular cytoplasm with intracytoplasmic mucin. The tissue fragments have areas of gland-like structure formation. Mitotic figures are identified.

The cytomorphologic changes described above are beyond the realm of reactive and are diagnostic of carcinoma. Pleomorphic adenomas show characteristic metachromatic stroma (on Diff-Quik staining) admixed with benign epithelial elements. This case proved to be a high-grade salivary duct carcinoma on excisional biopsy. Salivary duct carcinoma is a rare neoplasm that typically occurs in older men in Stensen's duct of the parotid. A cribriform architectural pattern with central comedo-like necrosis is often seen on cytology specimens. These features were not readily apparent in this case, so a less specific diagnosis is warranted.

References

1. Mukunyadzi P. Review of fine-needle aspiration cytology of salivary gland neoplasms, with emphasis on differential diagnosis. *AJCP*. 2002;118(suppl):S100–S115.
2. Stewart CJ, MacKenzie K, McGarry GW, Mowat A. Fine-needle aspiration cytology of salivary gland: a review of 341 cases. *Diagn Cytopathol*. 2000;22(3):139–146.

CASE

78

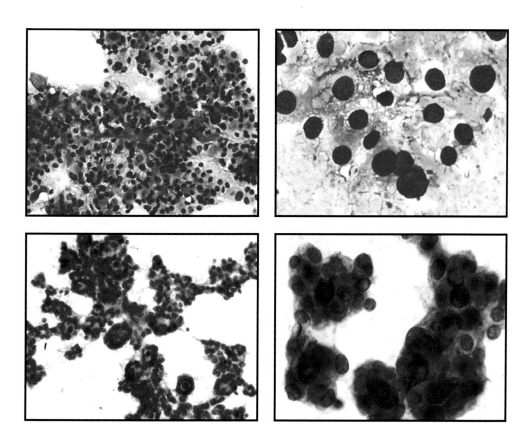

Clinical History

Fine needle aspiration (FNA) of a thyroid nodule in a 46-year-old female.

Choose the Best Diagnosis

a. Suspicious for a follicular neoplasm

b. Suspicious for a Hurthle cell neoplasm

c. Benign, consistent with an adenomatoid nodule

d. Benign, consistent with lymphocytic thyroiditis

e. Papillary thyroid carcinoma

ANSWER AND BRIEF DISCUSSION

e. Papillary Thyroid Carcinoma

These smears are extremely cellular and contain minimal colloid. The follicular cells are arranged in small fragments, some of which display microfollicular structures. There is moderate nuclear enlargement present.

Because of the abundance of follicular epithelium and the paucity of colloid, this FNA is most likely a neoplasm. The follicular cells contain moderately enlarged, round nuclei and are arranged in microfollicular structures. Because of these features, this lesion falls into the broad category of a follicular neoplasm; however, there are several clues present that this is not a follicular adenoma or a follicular carcinoma. Focally, there is striking nuclear enlargement present. Many of the nuclei contain a fine powdery chromatin that is more consistent with a papillary carcinoma than a follicular neoplasm. In addition, there are prominent longitudinal grooves and occasional inclusions present in many of the nuclei. Consequently, this is most consistent with a follicular variant of papillary carcinoma.

References

1. Cibas ES, Ali SZ. The Bethesda system for reporting thyroid cytopathology. *Thyroid: Official Journal of the American Thyroid Association*. 2009;19(11):1159–1165.
2. Baloch ZW, LiVolsi VA, Asa SL, et al. Diagnostic terminology and morphologic criteria for cytologic diagnosis of thyroid lesions: a synopsis of the National Cancer Institute thyroid fine-needle aspiration state of the science conference. *Diagn Cytopathol*. 2008;36(6):425–437.

CASE

79

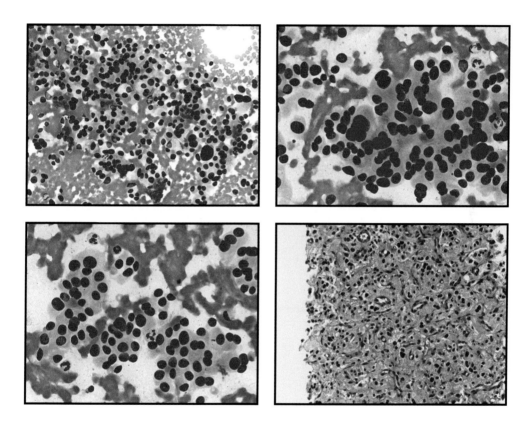

Clinical History

Fine needle aspiration (FNA) of a pelvic mass in a 35-year-old male, near the aortic arch.

Choose the Best Diagnosis

a. High-grade urothelial carcinoma

b. Renal cell carcinoma

c. Metastatic papillary thyroid carcinoma

d. Plasmacytoma

e. Paraganglioma

ANSWER AND BRIEF DISCUSSION

e. Paraganglioma

The smears are cellular and contain a monotonous population of cells. The cells have abundant granular cytoplasm and round to oval eccentrically placed nuclei. While the nuclei have smooth borders, there is dramatic anisonucleosis. Prominent nucleoli are not identified. The cells are present in discohesive groups. The neoplastic cells have similar features on the cell block preparation, where they are present in nests surrounding vessels, a feature not identified in the smear preparations.

While a Papanicolaou stain would have better demonstrated nuclear neuroendocrine features, the above findings are most consistent with paraganglioma among the possible choices. The cytomorphology is consistent with a neuroendocrine neoplasm, and if sampling is from an adrenal lesion, the differential diagnosis includes pheochromocytoma and adrenal cortical neoplasms. In this case, confirmatory immunostains for chromogranin and synaptophysin highlight chief cells, while S-100 protein would be positive in sustentacular cells. Paragangliomas are often vascular, which may result in abundant blood contamination with only rare tumor cells on FNA.

Reference

1. Rana RS, Dey P, Das A. Fine needle aspiration (FNA) cytology of extra-adrenal paragangliomas. *Cytopathology*. 1997;8(2):108–113.

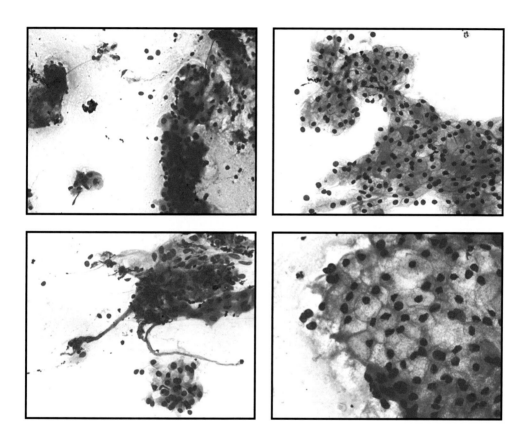

Clinical History

Fine needle aspiration of a parotid mass in a 27-year-old woman.

Choose the Best Diagnosis

    a. Mucoepidermoid carcinoma (MEC)

    b. Acinic cell carcinoma

    c. Metastatic renal cell carcinoma

    d. Pleomorphic adenoma

    e. Sialadenitis

ANSWER AND BRIEF DISCUSSION

a. Mucoepidermoid Carcinoma (MEC)

The aspirates are cellular and show predominantly cohesive epithelial cells. The majority of the cells have clear/vacuolated cytoplasm. There are cells in lesser quantities with thicker, metaplastic type cytoplasm. The nuclei are low grade without significant atypia.

This is a challenging case. The cellularity suggests a neoplastic process. The finding of multiple cell types is suggestive of MEC. MEC is notable for heterogeneity, and the epithelial component may be squamoid, mucinous, or of intermediate cell type. In this case, the clear/vacuolated cells represent mucinous cells, and the cells with more dense, metaplastic cytoplasm represent intermediate cells. An important differential to consider in cases of suspected low-grade MEC is sialadenitis or a retention cyst with squamous metaplasia. Sialadenitis is often cystic (like MEC) and can have foamy macrophages that simulate mucinous epithelium. The macrophages are more often singly dispersed, and finding mucinous cells in a tissue fragment supports an epithelial origin.

References

1. Stewart CJ, MacKenzie K, McGarry GW, Mowat A. Fine-needle aspiration cytology of salivary gland: a review of 341 cases. *Diagn Cytopathol.* 2000;22(3):139–146.
2. Mukunyadzi P. Review of fine-needle aspiration cytology of salivary gland neoplasms, with emphasis on differential diagnosis. *Am J Clin Pathol.* 2002;118(suppl):S100–S115.

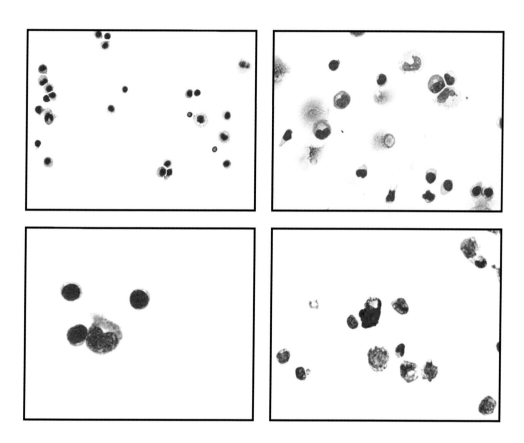

Clinical History

A 60-year-old female with headache and nuchal rigidity. Cerebrospinal fluid (CSF). Flow cytometry does not reveal a phenotypic abnormality.

Choose the Best Diagnosis

a. Changes consistent with Lyme meningitis

b. Hodgkin lymphoma

c. Toxoplasmosis

d. Malignant lymphoma

e. Metastatic melanoma

ANSWER AND BRIEF DISCUSSION

a. Changes Consistent With Lyme Meningitis

The CSF is more cellular than normal with a predominance of mononuclear cells. Rare atypical-appearing lymphocytes are present.

Acquisition of additional data was critical in discerning the etiology of the CSF findings. The patient did have a rash best described as erythema chronicum migrans. In addition, Lyme serology was positive for both IgG and IgM. Protein electrophoresis of the CSF would likely display oligoclonal banding.

Reference

1. Razavi-Encha F, Fleury-Feith J, Gherardi R, Bernaudin JF. Cytologic features of cerebrospinal fluid in lyme disease. *Acta Cytol.* 1987;31(4):439–440.

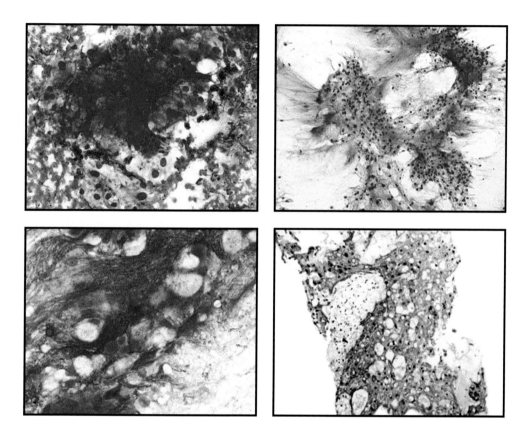

Clinical History

A 42-year-old man with sacral pain. Fine needle aspiration of the sacral mass. An S-100 protein immunostain is provided.

Choose the Best Diagnosis

    a. Chondrosarcoma

    b. Myxopapillary ependymoma

    c. Chordoma

    d. Cellular schwannoma

    e. Melanoma

ANSWER AND BRIEF DISCUSSION

c. Chordoma

Smears show fragments of intermediate to large polygonal cells with uniform, round nuclei embedded in a metachromatic fibrillar matrix. No significant nuclear pleomorphism or mitotic activity is appreciated. Closer inspection of the cells reveals some of them to be vacuolated.

This midline mass has a benign cytologic appearance and is most consistent with a chordoma. The vacuolated (physaliphorous) cells, cytokeratin, and S-100 protein positivity confirm this diagnosis. Chordomas affect males more commonly than females and tend to occur at the base of the skull, cervical region, and sacrum. Lesions of the sacrum may be difficult to identify radiologically, and treatment may be delayed as a result.

References

1. Walaas L, Kindblom LG. Fine-needle aspiration biopsy in the preoperative diagnosis of chordoma: a study of 17 cases with application of electron microscopic, histochemical, and immunocytochemical examination. *Hum Pathol*. 1991;22(1):22–28.
2. Finley JL, Silverman JF, Dabbs DJ, et al. Chordoma: diagnosis by fine-needle aspiration biopsy with histologic, immunocytochemical, and ultrastructural confirmation. *Diagn Cytopathol*. 1986;2(4):330–337.

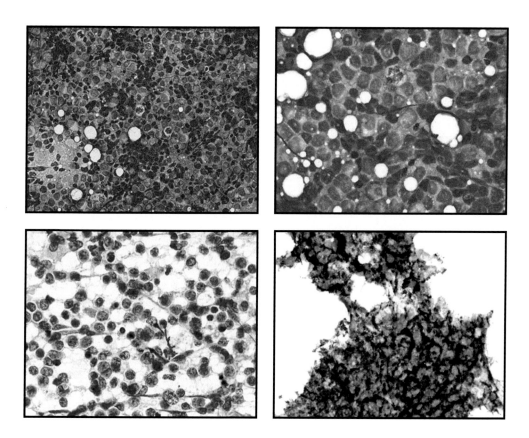

Clinical History

An 11-year-old with pelvic ramus fracture. Fine needle aspiration of the pelvic mass. Flow cytometry is negative for monoclonal lymphoid population. A CD99 immunostain is provided.

Choose the Best Diagnosis

a. Lymphoblastic lymphoma

b. Metastatic Wilms' tumor

c. Rhabdomyosarcoma

d. Ewing sarcoma/primitive neuroectodermal tumor (PNET)

e. Metastatic melanoma

ANSWER AND BRIEF DISCUSSION

d. Ewing Sarcoma/Primitive Neuroectodermal Tumor (PNET)

Smears contain confluent sheets of small round blue cells with a dimorphic population. Some are larger blastemic-appearing cells, while others are smaller and lymphocyte-like. There are numerous mitoses. No well-defined rosettes or tubules are seen.

The histology and age bring up the "small blue cell tumor" differential: lymphoma, rhabdomyosarcoma, Ewing/PNET, neuroblastoma, and Wilms' tumor. Immunophenotyping with markers such as myogenin, synaptophysin, CD45, CD79a, desmin, and O13 (CD99) can aid in the diagnosis. Cytogenetically, Ewing sarcoma displays t(11;22).

References

1. Lewis TB, Coffin CM, Bernard PS. Differentiating Ewing's sarcoma from other round blue cell tumors using a RT-PCR translocation panel on formalin-fixed paraffin-embedded tissues. *Mod Pathol.* 2007;20(3):397–404.
2. Renshaw AA, Perez-Atayde AR, Fletcher JA, Granter SR. Cytology of typical and atypical Ewing's sarcoma/PNET. *Am J Clin Pathol.* 1996;106(5):620–624.

CASE

84

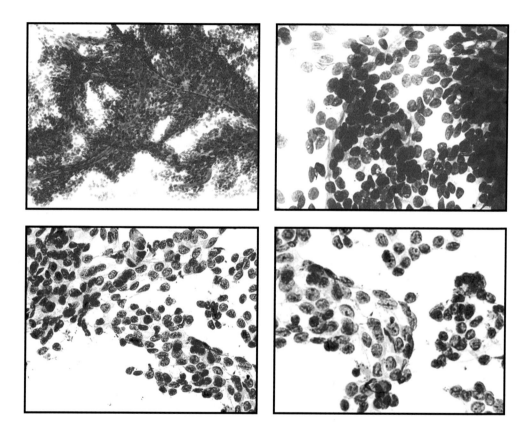

Clinical History

Fine needle aspiration of a liver mass in a 37-year-old woman with a history of a malignant neoplasm.

Choose the Best Diagnosis

a. Metastatic medullary thyroid carcinoma

b. Metastatic dysgerminoma

c. Metastatic lobular breast carcinoma

d. Metastatic granulosa cell tumor (GCT)

e. Metastatic colonic adenocarcinoma

ANSWER AND BRIEF DISCUSSION

d. Metastatic Granulosa Cell Tumor (GCT)

The aspirates are cellular and consist of a monotonous population of tumor cells with traversing capillaries. The nuclei are round to oval in shape, and there is only a small amount of wispy cytoplasm (and thus high N/C ratios). Careful examination of nuclear features in the Papanicolaou-stained material reveals pale staining chromatin with numerous longitudinal grooves and inconspicuous nucleoli. Significant mitotic activity was not appreciated.

This case is an excellent example of GCT. Papillary thyroid carcinoma should be considered because the nuclear features are so similar, but the finding of Call-Exner bodies and the lack of intranuclear inclusions makes GCT the most likely diagnosis. The other answer choices are not as likely, considering the described cytomorphology. GCTs are the most common ovarian sex cord stromal tumors and are extremely estrogenic to the point of causing postmenopausal bleeding in older patients and menorrhagia in younger women. Endometrial hyperplasia (and sometimes carcinoma) usually accompanies GCT. The tumors are also clinically unique in that they can recur long after initial diagnosis and resection (greater than 2-decade intervals have been reported). The tumor cells are immunoreactive for inhibin. The prognosis is relatively good with a nearly 90% 10-year survival rate.

Reference

1. Lal A, Bourtsos EP, Nayar R, DeFrias DV. Cytologic features of granulosa cell tumors in fluids and fine needle aspiration specimens. *Acta Cytol.* 2004;48(3):315–320.

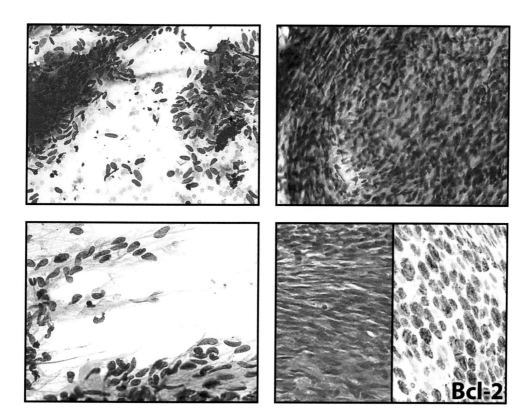

Clinical History

A 14-year-old girl with a large soft-tissue mass in the proximal calf with no bony involvement. Fine needle aspiration.

Choose the Best Diagnosis

a. Ewing sarcoma/primitive neuroectodermal tumor (PNET)

b. Synovial sarcoma

c. Schwannoma

d. Follicular lymphoma

e. Malignant melanoma

ANSWER AND BRIEF DISCUSSION

b. Synovial Sarcoma

The smears are very cellular and show numerous large fragments and scattered single cells. The architecture is vaguely fascicular and slightly disordered. At high power, these cells have a spindled appearance with a few intact elongated cells and many bare, hyperchromatic nuclei. Most of the nuclei are oval and plump to "cigar shaped" with fine chromatin and no nucleoli. No matrix or osteoid is identified in the background.

The biopsy shows a very darkly staining core of tissue with fascicles of spindle cells. These cells have a high N/C ratio, hyperchromatic nuclei, and fine to slightly grainy chromatin. Immunostain is positive for Bcl-2. The tumor is nonreactive for EMA, S-100 protein, and CD34 (not shown).

The hematoxylin and eosin (H&E) morphology of synovial sarcoma (monophasic in this material) is very characteristically hyperchromatic with plump spindled nuclei and very little cytoplasm. The positive Bcl-2 immunostain helps confirm this impression. The plump, hyperchromatic nuclei and high N/C ratios are more atypical than are usually seen in schwannomas.

Ewing sarcoma would be a clinical consideration given the patient's age and the site, and while Ewing/PNETs can be positive for Bcl-2, the morphology in this case is clearly not that of a small round blue cell tumor. Similarly, while follicular lymphomas typically have translocations involving Bcl-2 that cause its overexpression, the cytomorphology here is not lymphoid due to the predominance of spindle cells and the many cohesive fragments.

References

1. Akerman M, Willen H, Carlen B, Mandahl N, Mertens F. Fine needle aspiration (FNA) of synovial sarcoma--a comparative histological-cytological study of 15 cases, including immunohistochemical, electron microscopic and cytogenetic examination and DNA-ploidy analysis. *Cytopathol.* 1996;7(3):187–200.
2. Costa MJ, Campman SC, Davis RL, Howell LP. Fine-needle aspiration cytology of sarcoma: retrospective review of diagnostic utility and specificity. *Diagn Cytopathol.* 1996;15(1):23–32.

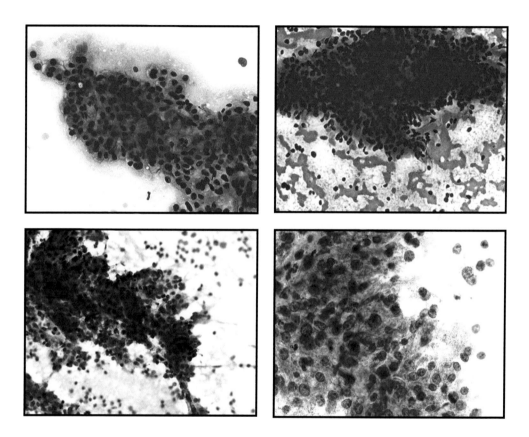

Clinical History

Fine needle aspiration of left clavicle in a 77-year-old female with a history of hepatocellular carcinoma.

Choose the Best Diagnosis

a. Osteosarcoma

b. Metastatic hepatocellular carcinoma (HCC)

c. Metastatic adenocarcinoma

d. Liposarcoma

e. Large cell lymphoma

ANSWER AND BRIEF DISCUSSION

b. Metastatic Hepatocellular Carcinoma (HCC)

The aspirate consists of numerous cohesive fragments of polygonal epithelial cells with increased N/C ratios and large round central nuclei. The chromatin is coarsely granular, and many of the cells have prominent nucleoli. Several naked nuclei are seen adjacent to the cohesive groups.

The described cytomorphologic features are consistent with metastatic carcinoma. Although soft-tissue malignancies should be considered, the cohesiveness and morphology of the cells favor an epithelial origin. The malignant polygonal cells are reminiscent of hepatocytes. Given the history, a diagnosis of metastatic HCC is rendered. A hepatocyte paraffin-1 immunostain is confirmatory.

Reference

1. Siddiqui MT, Saboorian MH, Gokaslan ST, Ashfaq R. Diagnostic utility of the HepPar1 antibody to differentiate hepatocellular carcinoma from metastatic carcinoma in fine-needle aspiration samples. *Cancer.* 2002;96(1):49–52.

CASE

87

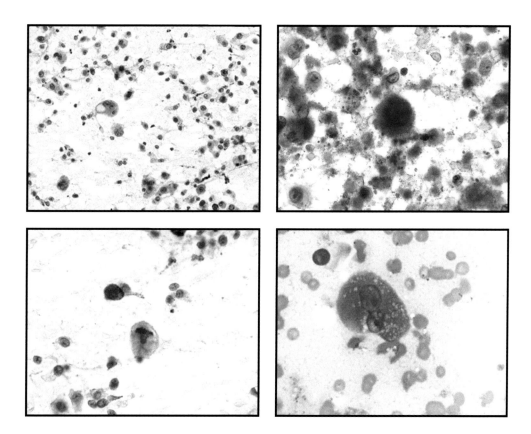

Clinical History

Fine needle aspiration of liver in a 52-year-old male with a history of melanoma and colonic adenocarcinoma.

Choose the Best Diagnosis

a. Giant cell hepatitis

b. Metastatic colonic adenocarcinoma

c. Hepatocellular carcinoma

d. Metastatic melanoma

e. Echinococcosis (hydatid cyst)

ANSWER AND BRIEF DISCUSSION

d. Metastatic Melanoma

The cellular aspirate consists of polygonal hepatocytes, blood, and large discohesive markedly atypical cells with coarse brown melanin granules. The nuclei of the atypical cells are round with multiple prominent nucleoli and macronucleoli. The melanin pigment obscures cytomorphologic detail in many of the cells. A characteristic binucleated cell with macronucleoli is noted in the Diff-Quik preparation. Frequent mitoses and abnormal mitoses are present.

The mentioned features are diagnostic of metastatic malignant melanoma. The presence of melanin pigment in the malignant cells essentially excludes all other diagnoses. Carcinomas would be more cohesive and less pleomorphic than malignant melanoma. Finally, giant cell hepatitis is a nonspecific reactive condition of the liver that sometimes occurs after a liver insult, most commonly in neonates.

Reference

1. Parwani AV, Chan TY, Mathew S, Ali SZ. Metastatic malignant melanoma in liver aspirate: cytomorphologic distinction from hepatocellular carcinoma. *Diagn Cytopathol.* 2004;30(4):247–50.

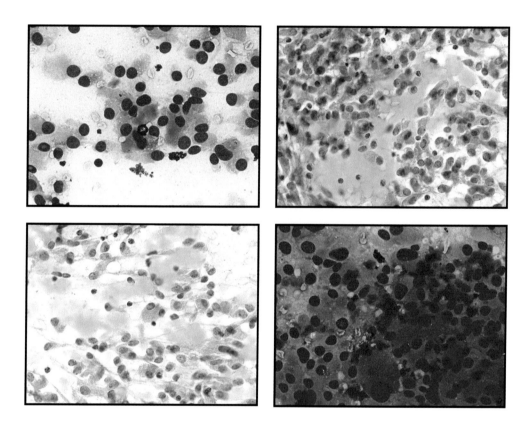

Clinical History

Fine needle aspiration of a 0.6-cm neck mass, level III, in a 41-year-old woman.

Choose the Best Diagnosis

    a. Medullary thyroid carcinoma

    b. Paraganglioma

    c. Metastatic renal cell carcinoma

    d. Metastatic melanoma

    e. Oncocytoma

ANSWER AND BRIEF DISCUSSION

a. Medullary Thyroid Carcinoma

The smears are cellular, containing a monotonous population of discohesive cells. The cells have a plasmacytoid appearance, with abundant granular cytoplasm; some granules are red. The chromatin has a "salt-and-pepper" appearance, identified most readily on Papanicolaou-stained smears. There is minimal nuclear pleomorphism; the nuclei are round and without prominent nucleoli. Amorphous extracellular material is readily identified on both Pap stain and Diff-Quik.

The differential diagnosis of a neck mass is broad, given the number of tissues that may be present at the site (salivary gland, lymph node, thyroid, etc.). In this case, the neuroendocrine features (chromatin pattern, eccentric regular round nuclei, and discohesive cells) favor either medullary thyroid carcinoma or paraganglioma from the choices presented. However, the presence of amorphous material (presumably amyloid) strongly suggests medullary thyroid carcinoma, which may be metastatic to a lymph node or primary to the thyroid depending on the sampling. Without a history, definitive diagnosis requires staining with calcitonin (tumor cells) or Congo red (amyloid). Positive staining for chromogranin and synaptophysin does not exclude paraganglioma in the absence of amyloid.

References

1. Cibas ES, Ali SZ. The Bethesda system for reporting thyroid cytopathology. *Thyroid: Official Journal of the American Thyroid Association.* 2009;19(11):1159–1165.
2. Baloch ZW, Cibas ES, Clark DP, et al. The National Cancer Institute thyroid fine needle aspiration state of the science conference: a summation. *CytoJournal.* 2008;5:6.

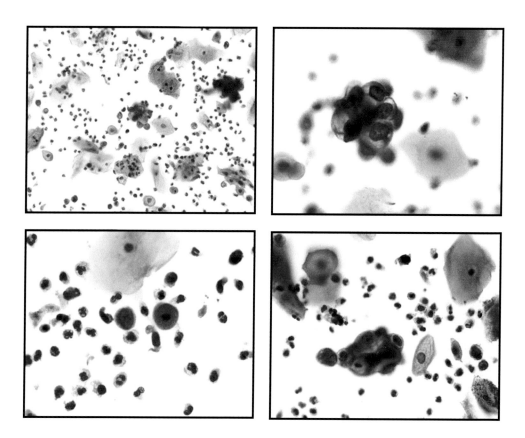

Clinical History

Liquid-based Pap test (SurePath) in a 49-year-old female.

Choose the Best Diagnosis

a. Negative for intraepithelial lesion and malignancy, changes secondary to intrauterine device (IUD)

b. Endometrial adenocarcinoma

c. Microglandular hyperplasia

d. High-grade squamous intraepithelial lesion

e. Tubal metaplasia

ANSWER AND BRIEF DISCUSSION

b. Endometrial Adenocarcinoma

The Pap test consists of rare fragments and single atypical glandular cells in a background of squamous cells and acute inflammation. The atypical cells are rounded and have increased N/C ratios with irregular nuclear contours and clumped chromatin with some discernible nucleoli. Mitotic figures were identified.

The features noted previously warrant tissue studies. The morphology of the atypical cells favors an endometrial origin. In perimenopausal and postmenopausal women, the presence of atypical endometrial cells is especially worrisome. IUDs may cause clustering of atypical hypervacuolated endocervical cells or exfoliate single atypical endometrial cells that can mimic carcinoma. One should be careful when diagnosing adenocarcinoma in a patient wearing an IUD. In this case, atypical glandular cells (AGC) would be a reasonable diagnosis as well. Endometrial carcinoma was diagnosed on subsequent biopsy.

References

1. Solomon D, Nayar R. *The Bethesda System for Reporting Cervical Cytology: Definitions, Criteria, and Explanatory Notes.* 2nd ed. New York, NY: Springer; 2006:123–156.
2. Sherman ME, Dasgupta A, Schiffman M, Nayar R, Solomon D: The Bethesda Interobserver Reproducibility Study (BIRST): a web-based assessment of the Bethesda 2001 System for classifying cervical cytology. *Cancer.* 2007;111(1):15–25.

CASE

90

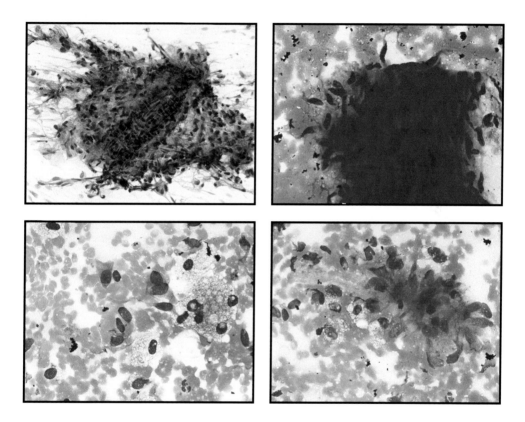

Clinical History

Fine needle aspiration (FNA) of a 2.2-cm rapidly growing posterior knee mass in a 17-year-old male.

Choose the Best Diagnosis

a. Giant cell tumor of tendon sheath

b. Melanoma

c. Nodular fasciitis (NF)

d. High-grade sarcoma

e. Tuberculoma

ANSWER AND BRIEF DISCUSSION

c. Nodular Fasciitis (NF)

The smears contain spindle cells present both in fragments and as single cells. For a soft-tissue mass, the smear is relatively cellular. Even though there is mild nuclear pleomorphism, the chromatin is bland, and prominent nucleoli are not seen. Mitotic figures and necrosis are not identified. In some areas, the cells are associated with a delicate myxoid-appearing matrix. The background also contains a mixture of inflammatory cells, including histiocytes with multinucleation.

NF is seen in children and young adults and presents as a rapidly growing subcutaneous lesion. Some lesions demonstrate striking pleomorphism and mitotic activity, which may result in the initial impression of a malignant process. The myxoid background may also suggest other myxoid lesions, such as myxofibrosarcoma. The nuclei are too bland to represent a high-grade sarcoma, though synovial sarcoma may enter the differential. The spindle cell morphology is not characteristic of giant cell tumor of the tendon sheath. While melanoma can present with spindle cell morphology, it is not associated with matrix material. Because these lesions often spontaneously regress, care must be taken to not overcall these lesions on FNA. Correlation with clinical history and/or core biopsy material is required for a definitive diagnosis.

Reference

1. Layfield LJ, Anders KH, Glasgow BJ, Mirra JM. Fine-needle aspiration of primary soft-tissue lesions. *Arch Path Lab Med.* 1986;110(5):420–424.

CASE
91

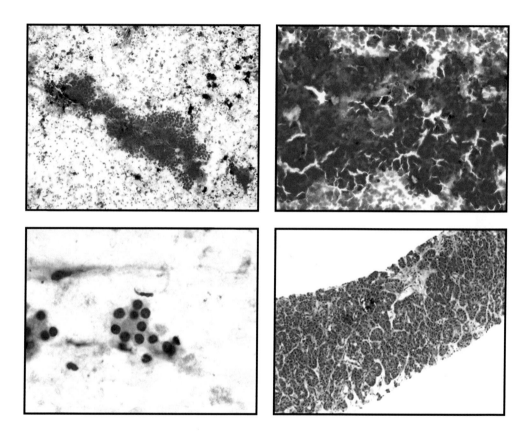

Clinical History

Fine needle aspiration (FNA) and core biopsy of a multiloculated mass involving peripancreatic soft tissues, perirenal tissue, and the retroperitoneum in a 52-year-old man who presents with obstructive jaundice and weight loss.

Choose the Best Diagnosis

a. Acinar cell carcinoma

b. Lymphoepithelial cyst

c. Pseudocyst

d. Pancreatic neuroendocrine tumor

e. Adenocarcinoma

ANSWER AND BRIEF DISCUSSION

c. Pseudocyst

The smears are hypocellular and show cells with benign-appearing nuclei and acinar arrangements. Pigmented material and pigment-laden macrophages are present in the background. The needle core biopsy directed in the same area of the cellular passes showed completely normal pancreatic tissue.

This was a challenging case requiring close communication with the clinical team and radiologists. This patient's presentation was very worrisome for a malignant process, and the initial radiographic impression was that the lesion was neoplastic. The first few passes were extremely cellular, but the Pap-stained material and the biopsy indicated normal pancreatic sampling. The needle was directed at the lesion, not the pancreas, but review of the scans after the FNA showed altered anatomy secondary to the multiloculated cystic lesion. The FNA was signed out descriptively, and nonneoplastic considerations were raised in the differential.

The patient had an open biopsy of the cyst wall, which showed inflamed fibrous tissue without associated epithelium and pigment-laden macrophages consistent with a pseudocyst.

References

1. Gonzalez Obeso E, Murphy E, Brugge W, Deshpande V. Pseudocyst of the pancreas: the role of cytology and special stains for mucin. *Cancer.* 2009;117:101–107.
2. Pitman MB, Deshpande V. Endoscopic ultrasound-guided fine needle aspiration cytology of the pancreas: a morphological and multimodal approach to the diagnosis of solid and cystic mass lesions. *Cytopathol.* 2007;18:331–347.

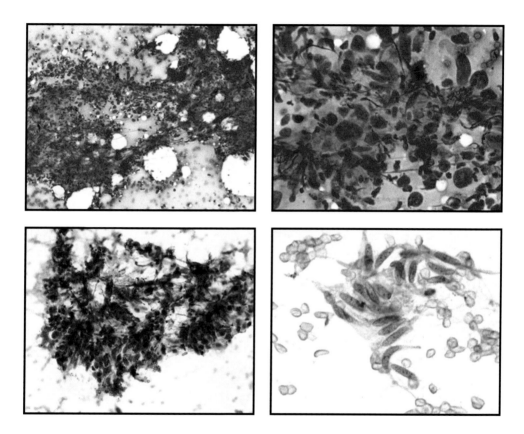

Clinical History

A 69-year-old female with a mass in the left thigh adjacent to a scar. Fine needle aspiration.

Choose the Best Diagnosis

a. Nodular fasciitis (NF)

b. Dermatofibrosarcoma protuberans (DFSP)

c. Melanoma

d. High-grade sarcoma, not otherwise specified (NOS)

e. Adenocarcinoma

ANSWER AND BRIEF DISCUSSION

d. High-Grade Sarcoma, NOS

This is a markedly abnormal specimen containing large numbers of enlarged pleomorphic cells. The cells are arranged singly and in small tissue fragments. They have a moderate amount of delicate cytoplasm. Closer inspection reveals a plump spindled morphology with blunted nuclei.

The cytomorphologic features are enough to classify this as a high-grade malignancy, but there are some clues to eliminate other possibilities. No myxoid background is present (as is seen in NF), and no pigment is present as may be seen in melanoma. There is no suggestion of the storiform pattern as seen in DFSP, leaving high-grade sarcoma the best choice. This patient had a history of leiomyosarcoma, and this neoplasm was positive for actin, but negative for S-100 protein (not shown), consistent with recurrent leiomyosarcoma.

Reference

1. Domanski HA, Akerman M, Rissler P, Gustafson P. Fine-needle aspiration of soft tissue leiomyosarcoma: an analysis of the most common cytologic findings and the value of ancillary techniques. *Diagn Cytopathol.* 2006;34:597–604.

CASE

93

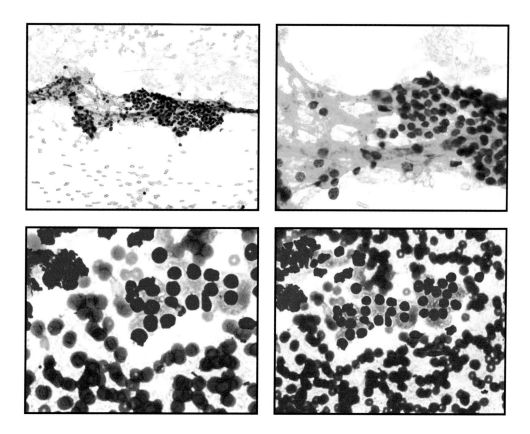

Clinical History

This fine needle aspiration (FNA) is from a 45-year-old man with a 2.3-cm lesion in the right lower pole of the thyroid.

Choose the Best Diagnosis

a. Suspicious for a follicular neoplasm

b. Papillary thyroid carcinoma

c. Suspicious for a Hurthle cell neoplasm

d. Parathyroid tissue

e. Benign, consistent with an adenomatoid nodule

ANSWER AND BRIEF DISCUSSION

d. Parathyroid Tissue

The smears show clusters of small, monomorphic cells with several naked nuclei in an otherwise clean background. The nuclei have a "salt-and-pepper" appearance and appear to form microfollicles in some areas. This patient was diagnosed with a parathyroid adenoma after excision of the mass. His clinical history included elevated serum calcium and parathyroid hormone (PTH) levels.

The nuclei of parathyroid cells are usually round to oval and smaller than red blood cells. Larger, pleomorphic nuclei can be identified, even in benign lesions. Nucleoli are usually inconspicuous. Cells may have fine red secretory granules (best seen on Diff-Quik stain). Cells can also form microfollicles. A PTH level can be obtained on the aspirated tissue to confirm the diagnosis; immunostaining for PTH can also help.

It can be quite difficult to differentiate parathyroid tissue from thyroid on FNA, and lesions can coexist in 10% of cases. The presence of colloid and macrophages favors thyroid origin (as well as staining for thyroglobulin), and thyroid lesions tend to have fewer naked nuclei, coarse chromatin, and larger cells overall. It may also be quite difficult to differentiate other neuroendocrine tumors such as paraganglioma and medullary thyroid carcinoma from FNA alone.

References

1. Cibas ES, Ali SZ. The Bethesda system for reporting thyroid cytopathology. *Thyroid.* 2009;19: 1159–1165.
2. Baloch ZW, Cibas ES, Clark DP, et al. The National Cancer Institute thyroid fine needle aspiration state of the science conference: a summation. *Cytojournal.* 2008;5:6.

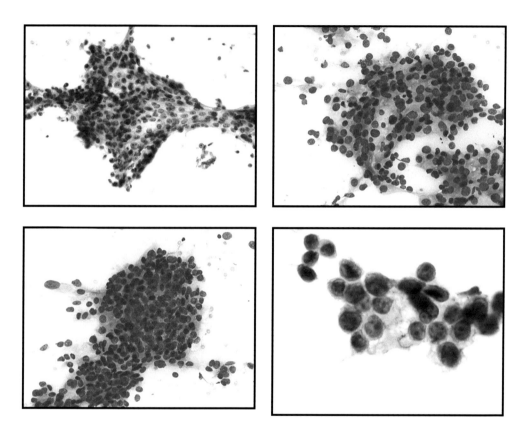

Clinical History

A 64-year-old female with a history of mastectomy now with a 2-cm thyroid nodule. Fine needle aspiration of the thyroid.

Choose the Best Diagnosis

a. Papillary thyroid carcinoma

b. Medullary thyroid carcinoma

c. Anaplastic thyroid carcinoma

d. Metastatic carcinoma consistent with breast primary

e. Suspicious for a follicular neoplasm

ANSWER AND BRIEF DISCUSSION

d. Metastatic Carcinoma Consistent With Breast Primary

The aspirate shows fragments of malignant epithelial cells with enlarged, pleomorphic nuclei. The cells have irregular nuclear contours and clumped chromatin. Some of the cells have prominent nucleoli. The background consists of colloid, blood, and benign thyroid epithelium.

Secondary carcinoma of the thyroid gland is relatively uncommon. Metastatic disease of the thyroid is found in about 10% of patients dying of malignant tumors. Several case reports and small studies have implicated many primary tumors in secondary malignancy of the thyroid. Rarely, metastatic disease of the thyroid may simulate clinically a primary thyroid neoplasm. In this case, the cytomorphologic features are diagnostic of malignancy. The morphology, however, is not consistent with thyroid epithelial origin. Anaplastic carcinoma of the thyroid typically yields a cellular aspirate with bizarre giant cells or spindled cells. Medullary carcinoma should have a salt-and-pepper chromatin pattern, typically without nucleoli. Immunostains can be important in distinguishing primary from metastatic carcinoma of the thyroid, but one should remember that diffusion of thyroglobulin and absorption by metastatic tumor cells can occur. In this case, subsequent imaging studies revealed metastatic disease in the liver, and the decision was made to not resect the thyroid gland.

References

1. Cibas ES, Ali SZ. The Bethesda system for reporting thyroid cytopathology. *Thyroid*. 2009;19: 1159–1165.
2. Baloch ZW, Cibas ES, Clark DP, et al. The National Cancer Institute thyroid fine needle aspiration state of the science conference: a summation. *Cytojournal*. 2008;5:6.

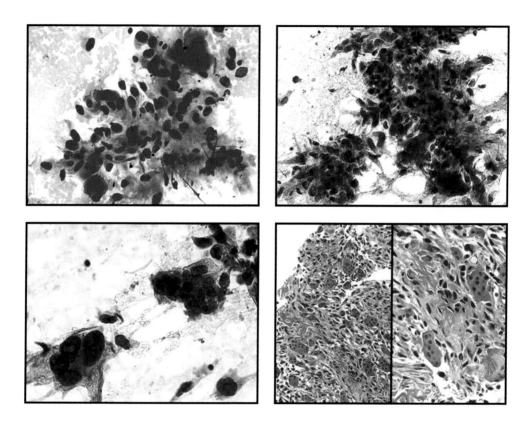

Clinical History

A 15-year-old boy with lesion of right tibia and soft tissue of right calf. Radiographic imaging shows a lesion in the diaphysis. A benign lesion is favored with a differential diagnosis including osteofibrous dysplasia. Fine needle aspiration (FNA).

Choose the Best Diagnosis

a. Fibrosarcoma

b. Chondrosarcoma

c. Osteosarcoma

d. Osteoid osteoma

e. Myositis ossificans

ANSWER AND BRIEF DISCUSSION

c. Osteosarcoma

The fine needle aspirate is abundantly cellular, composed of aggregates of polygonal cells as well as spindled cells. Closer examination reveals several multinucleated giant cells, some with small bland nuclei (osteoclast giant cells) and others with larger, atypical nuclei (pleomorphic giant cells). Pink fibrillar material is present between cells with no definitive osteoid formation. The cell block reveals a collection of giant cells in a background of oval and plasmacytoid malignant osteoblasts, interwoven with fibrillar osteoid material.

The presence of spindle cells with delicate cytoplasm radiating from the nucleus suggests a sarcomatous process. This finding, in addition to the identification of pleomorphic and atypical giant cells, in the context of plasmacytoid polygonal cells, suggests osteosarcoma. There is very little matrix material on the aspirate. However, there is irregular osteoid material on the cell block, which is consistent with an osteoid-forming sarcoma.

Although the presence of atypical spindle cells raises the differential of sarcoma, osteosarcoma is difficult to diagnose on FNA in the absence of osteoid. The amount of osteoid on an aspirate varies considerably and is often scant or focal. In some cases, osteosarcomas may show chondroid matrix (chondroblastic osteosarcoma) or fibroid matrix (fibrosarcoma-like high-grade osteosarcoma), raising the possibility of a chondrosarcoma or fibrosarcoma. In these cases, a reaspiration or core biopsy may be helpful in establishing a definitive diagnosis.

Osteosarcoma is the most common primary tumor of the bone, whereas soft-tissue osteosarcomas are comparatively rare. Bone osteosarcomas usually occur in younger patients and most frequently occur in the distal femur, upper tibia, upper humerus, or vertebra. They are commonly in the metaphysis of the long bones, though involvement of almost all skeletal sites has been described. In this case, the diaphyseal location led to a benign radiographic impression.

References

1. Dodd LG, Scully SP, Cothran RL, Harrelson JM. Utility of fine-needle aspiration in the diagnosis of primary osteosarcoma. *Diagn Cytopathol*. 2002;27:350–353.
2. Bommer KK, Ramzy I, Mody D. Fine-needle aspiration biopsy in the diagnosis and management of bone lesions: a study of 450 cases. *Cancer*. 1997;81:148–156.

CASE

96

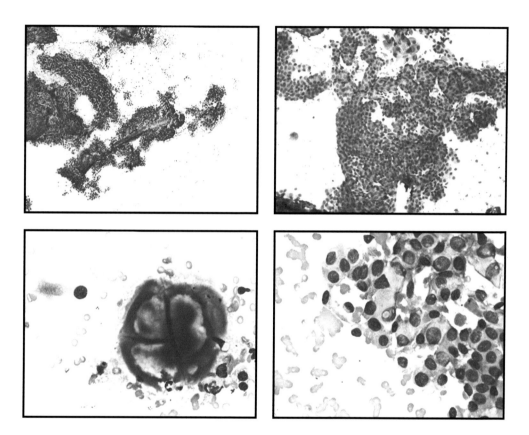

Clinical History

Thyroid fine needle aspiration in a 41-year-old male.

Choose the Best Diagnosis

    a. Suspicious for a follicular neoplasm

    b. Papillary thyroid carcinoma (PTC)

    c. Hashimoto thyroiditis

    d. Adenomatoid nodule

    e. Medullary thyroid carcinoma

ANSWER AND BRIEF DISCUSSION

b. Papillary Thyroid Carcinoma (PTC)

Numerous papillary epithelial fragments are appreciated from low power in this cellular aspirate. Closer inspection of the cells reveals crowded, enlarged nuclei with nuclear grooves and numerous intranuclear inclusions. Psammoma bodies are also identified.

This is a relatively straightforward case of PTC. The cellularity of the aspirate and architecture of the tissue fragments are concerning. The nuclear features appreciated at high power confirm the diagnosis of PTC.

References

1. Cibas ES, Ali SZ. The Bethesda system for reporting thyroid cytopathology. *Thyroid*. 2009;19: 1159–1165.
2. Baloch ZW, Cibas ES, Clark DP, et al. The National Cancer Institute thyroid fine needle aspiration state of the science conference: a summation. *Cytojournal*. 2008;5:6.

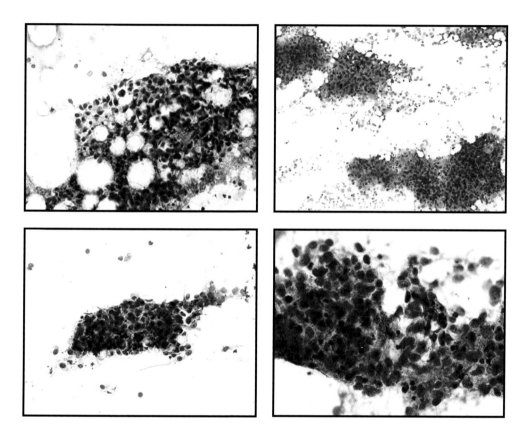

Clinical History

A 39-year-old male with nontender nodule in left neck with overlying scar. Fine needle aspiration of soft tissue mass.

Choose the Best Diagnosis

a. Granulation tissue with hemorrhage

b. High-grade sarcoma

c. Nodular fasciitis

d. Metastatic malignant melanoma

e. Granulomatous inflammation

ANSWER AND BRIEF DISCUSSION

d. Metastatic Malignant Melanoma

Smears from this aspirate are quite cellular, with sheets of spindled and epithelioid cells. These cells exhibit marked nuclear pleomorphism and nucleoli, and closer examination reveals cytoplasmic pigment.

This case emphasizes the protean nature of recurrent/metastatic melanoma. It can be a deceptive malignancy, especially when the history is remote or even unreported. Always keep this entity somewhere in your differential.

Reference

1. Perry MD, Gore M, Seigler HF, Johnston WW. Fine needle aspiration biopsy of metastatic melanoma. A morphologic analysis of 174 cases. *Acta Cytol.* 1986;30:385–396.

CASE

98

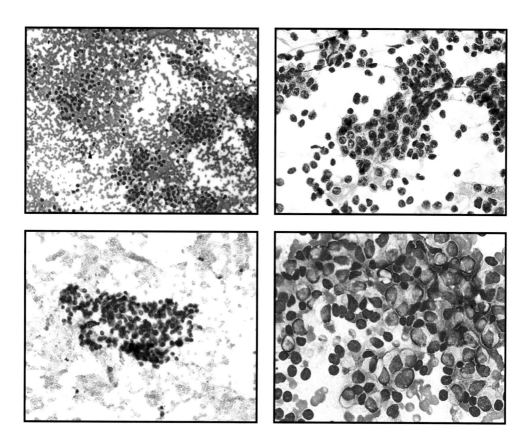

Clinical History

An 81-year-old male with liver lesion on CT. Ultrasound-guided fine needle aspiration.

Choose the Best Diagnosis

    a. Metastatic neuroendocrine tumor

    b. Bile duct hamartoma

    c. Metastatic adenocarcinoma

    d. Small cell carcinoma

    e. Hepatocellular carcinoma

ANSWER AND BRIEF DISCUSSION

a. Metastatic Neuroendocrine Tumor

Smears from this needle aspirate are cellular, nearly devoid of normal-appearing hepato-cytes, and quite suspicious for malignancy. Sheets and loose groups of cells have a monot-onous, plasmacytoid appearance. The nuclei are uniform and round with coarse, speckled chromatin. Ancillary special stains reveal positivity for cytokeratin as well as chromogranin.

The cytomorphologic features best fit a neuroendocrine tumor rather than an adenocar-cinoma. Small cell carcinoma may be a consideration, but the degree of nuclear pleomor-phism, lack of nuclear molding, and level of hyperchromasia do not reach the threshold for this diagnosis.

Reference

1. Nicholson SA, Ryan MR. A review of cytologic findings in neuroendocrine carcinomas including carcinoid tumors with histologic correlation. *Cancer*. 2000;90:148–161.

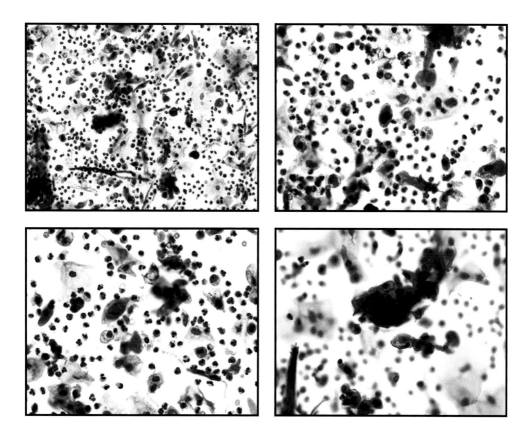

Clinical History

A 74-year-old male with hematuria and dysuria. Voided urine.

Choose the Best Diagnosis

a. High-grade urothelial carcinoma with squamous differentiation

b. Stone atypia

c. Cystitis glandularis

d. Malakoplakia

e. Candida changes

ANSWER AND BRIEF DISCUSSION

a. High-Grade Urothelial Carcinoma With Squamous Differentiation

This voided urine is quite cellular, with a background of acute inflammation. There are numerous admixed atypical cells that exhibit nuclear pleomorphism, hyperchromasia, and varying degrees of squamous differentiation.

Although the presence of stones may inflict significant cytologic atypia, this degree of atypia in concert with the cytoplasmic squamous differentiation favors the diagnosis of malignancy. Acute inflammation is present, but the lack of metaplastic glandular cells excludes the diagnosis of cystitis glandularis. Malakoplakia would exhibit a background of granulomatous inflammation and possibly Michaelis-Gutmann bodies.

References

1. Hattori M, Nishimura Y, Toyonaga M, Kakinuma H, Matsumoto K, Ohbu M. Cytological significance of abnormal squamous cells in urinary cytology. *Diagn Cytopathol.* 2012;40:798–803.
2. Owens CL, Ali SZ. Atypical squamous cells in exfoliative urinary cytology: clinicopathologic correlates. *Diagn Cytopathol.* 2005;33:394–398.

CASE

100

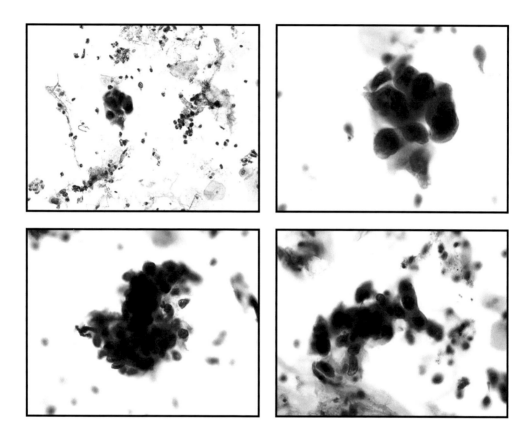

Clinical History

A 38-year-old with abnormal colposcopy. Liquid-based Pap test (SurePath).

Choose the Best Diagnosis

a. Atypical squamous cells of undetermined significance

b. High-grade squamous intraepithelial lesion (HSIL)

c. Low-grade squamous intraepithelial lesion

d. Reactive epithelial changes

e. Atypical glandular cells

ANSWER AND BRIEF DISCUSSION

b. High-Grade Squamous Intraepithelial Lesion (HSIL)

The slide shows a relatively clean background. Hyperchromatic crowded group of squamous cells are present. The cells have pleomorphic nuclei with irregular borders. No evidence of invasion is seen.

Concurrent colposcopic biopsy revealed HSIL. Once HSIL is identified, careful examination of the slide should be undertaken to determine whether additional related lesions are present, such as glandular involvement of HSIL or adenocarcinoma in situ.

References

1. Sherman ME, Dasgupta A, Schiffman M, Nayar R, Solomon D. The Bethesda Interobserver Reproducibility Study (BIRST): a web-based assessment of the Bethesda 2001 System for classifying cervical cytology. *Cancer.* 2007;111:15–25.
2. Solomon D, Nayar R. *The Bethesda System for Reporting Cervical Cytology: Definitions, Criteria, and Explanatory Notes.* 2nd ed. New York, NY: Springer; 2006:67–88.

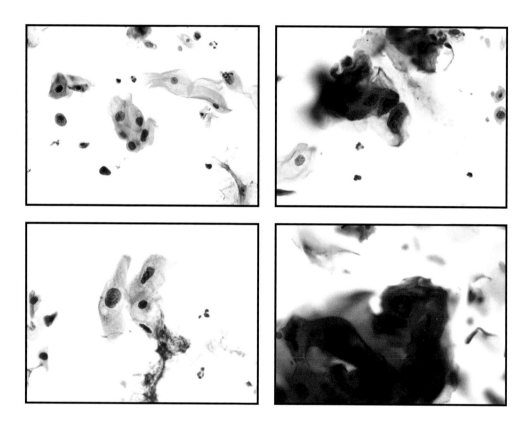

Anal smear in a 42-year-old man. SurePath.

    a. Anal intraepithelial neoplasm, grade I (AIN I)

    b. Reactive epithelial changes

    c. Anal intraepithelial neoplasm, grade III (AIN III)

    d. Atypical squamous cells of undetermined significance

    e. Squamous cell carcinoma

ANSWER AND BRIEF DISCUSSION

c. Anal Intraepithelial Neoplasm, Grade III (AIN III)

The smear shows dysplastic squamous cells with enlarged hyperchromatic nuclei, irregular nuclear contours, and a moderate amount of excessively keratinized cytoplasm. The background contains patchy areas of acute inflammation.

The described features are well beyond reactive or even low-grade dysplasia and are consistent with AIN III. There are occasional cells seen in the background, more suggestive of AIN I.

References

1. Darragh TM, Winkler B. Anal cancer and cervical cancer screening: key differences. *Cancer Cytopathol.* 2011;119:5–19.
2. Sherman ME, Dasgupta A, Schiffman M, Nayar R, Solomon D. The Bethesda Interobserver Reproducibility Study (BIRST): a web-based assessment of the Bethesda 2001 System for classifying cervical cytology. *Cancer.* 2007;111:15–25.

CASE

102

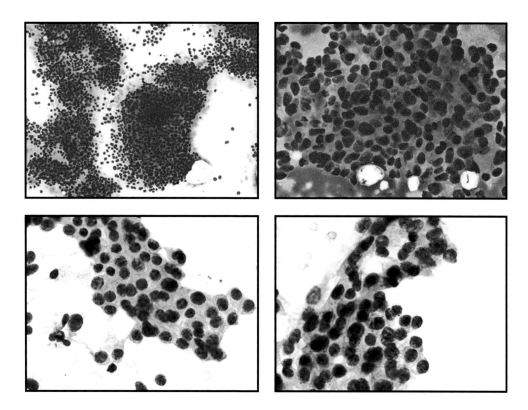

Clinical History

Hepatic fine needle aspiration in a 62-year-old man with multiple mass lesions of the liver.

Choose the Best Diagnosis

    a. Hepatocellular carcinoma

    b. Intrahepatic cholangiocarcinoma

    c. Metastatic adenocarcinoma consistent with colonic primary

    d. Metastatic carcinoid tumor

    e. Hepatic adenoma

ANSWER AND BRIEF DISCUSSION

d. Metastatic Carcinoid Tumor

The cellular aspirates show fragments and individual cells with round, monomorphic nuclei, high N/C ratios, and granular to speckled chromatin. The background is relatively clean, showing only scant blood.

The described nuclear features are typical of carcinoid tumor. Gastrointestinal carcinoid tumors that metastasize to the liver can cause vasomotor disturbances and intestinal hyper-motility owing to the release of secretory products into the systemic circulation. Clinically, this patient has carcinoid syndrome. The core biopsy showed a nested arrangement, and immunohistochemical stains were reactive for chromogranin and synaptophysin, proving the neuroendocrine origin of the cells.

Reference

1. Collins BT, Cramer HM. Fine needle aspiration cytology of carcinoid tumors. *Acta Cytol.* 1996;40:695–707.

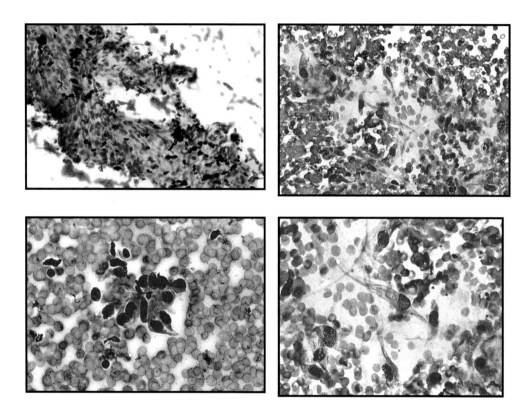

Clinical History

Fine needle aspiration (FNA) of a right inguinal lymph node in a 33-year-old man with acquired immune deficiency syndrome (AIDS) and inguinal lymphadenopathy.

Choose the Best Diagnosis

a. Nondiagnostic FNA

b. Lymphoid hyperplasia with granulomatous features

c. Kaposi sarcoma (KS)

d. Malignant peripheral nerve sheath tumor (MPNST)

e. Metastatic melanoma

ANSWER AND BRIEF DISCUSSION

c. Kaposi Sarcoma (KS)

The hypocellular smears contain scattered tissue fragments and individual spindle cells in a background of abundant blood. The nuclei are oval to elongated, and some of the cells have fibrillar cytoplasm. Scattered naked nuclei are present. Lymph node components were present in other fields (not shown).

The findings are consistent with disseminated KS. KS is a rare tumor, but is the most common sarcoma in patients with AIDS. Current evidence has implicated human herpes virus 8 as the causative agent. KS, unlike most sarcomas, frequently disseminates to lymph nodes. Although tumors of neural origin should be considered in the differential of spindle cell lesions, MPNSTs would tend to have higher grade nuclei and sometimes background necrosis. Although scattered neutrophils are present, they are simply a component of the background blood. Clinically, this patient has multiple KS lesions present on his extremities noted at the time of the FNA. Immunostains for vascular markers (CD31, CD34) are positive on the material in the cell block.

Reference

1. Hales M, Bottles K, Miller T, Donegan E, Ljung BM. Diagnosis of Kaposi's sarcoma by fine-needle aspiration biopsy. *Am J Clin Pathol.* 1987;88:20–25.

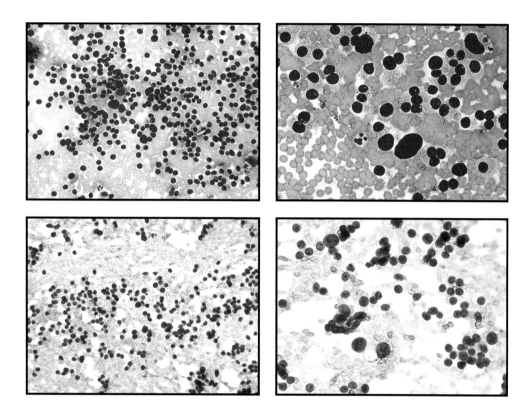

Clinical History

A 52-year-old woman who relates a history of thyroidectomy but could not recall the final diagnosis. Fine needle aspiration of mass in thyroid bed.

Choose the Best Diagnosis

a. Ectopic thyroid tissue

b. Medullary thyroid carcinoma

c. Suspicious for a Hurthle cell neoplasm

d. Suspicious for a follicular neoplasm

e. Papillary thyroid carcinoma

ANSWER AND BRIEF DISCUSSION

b. Medullary Thyroid Carcinoma

Numerous loosely cohesive cells having lymphoplasmacytoid features are seen. The nuclei are round and have a characteristic "salt-and-pepper" appearance.

Medullary thyroid carcinoma is characterized by neoplastic neuroendocrine cells with a distinctive finely granular chromatin pattern. While cases of medullary thyroid carcinoma may have Hurthloid and spindle cells, proportions vary from case to case, and the lymphoplasmacytoid population predominates here. Review of the original thyroidectomy material from an outside hospital confirmed the initial diagnosis of medullary thyroid carcinoma.

References

1. Baloch ZW, Cibas ES, Clark DP, et al. The National Cancer Institute thyroid fine needle aspiration state of the science conference: a summation. *Cytojournal.* 2008;5:6.
2. Cibas ES, Ali SZ. The Bethesda system for reporting thyroid cytopathology. *Thyroid.* 2009;19: 1159–1165.

CASE
105

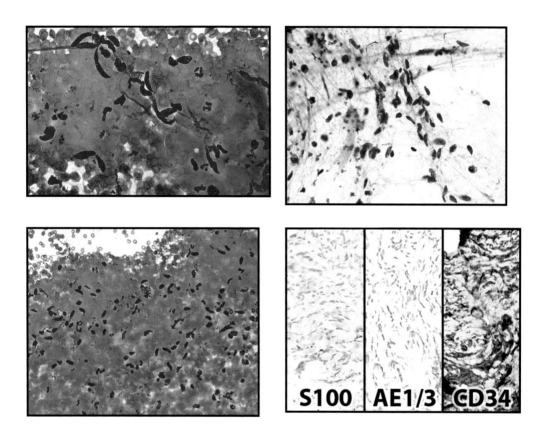

Clinical History

An 84-year-old man with a 4-cm anterior mediastinal mass on routine follow-up. Fine needle aspiration.

Choose the Best Diagnosis

a. Leiomyoma

b. Solitary fibrous tumor (SFT)

c. Myxoma

d. Schwannoma

e. High-grade pleomorphic sarcoma

ANSWER AND BRIEF DISCUSSION

b. Solitary Fibrous Tumor (SFT)

A low-power view shows fragments of cells in a clean background. Closer examination reveals spindled cells in loosely cohesive aggregates with bland tapered nuclei and wispy cytoplasm. The nuclei are oval in shape and regular in outline, with even chromatin. These clusters are admixed in a background of delicate vasculature. Stains for S-100 protein and AE1/3 are negative, while CD34 is positive.

SFTs are bland mesenchymal tumors that are usually small and well demarcated. They most commonly occur in the pleura, but have been reported to involve the head and neck, back, orbit, groin, and buttock.

Histologically, these lesions are composed of fascicles of spindled cells, raising the differential diagnosis of other spindle cell lesions such as leiomyomas, fibromatosis, gastrointestinal stromal tumor (GIST), melanoma, and MFH. SFTs have alternating areas of cellularity and stromal sclerosis, with no polarity. Fibromatosis has bland spindled cells with bipolar cytoplasmic processes sometimes oriented in a "stream of fish" pattern. Leiomyomas have blunt ended nuclei with perinuclear vacuoles. Schwannomas and neurofibromas have comma-shaped nuclei. GISTs typically display epithelioid areas as well as spindle cell areas. The lack of cytologic atypia would be unusual for melanoma or MFH.

References

1. Clayton AC, Salomao DR, Keeney GL, Nascimento AG. Solitary fibrous tumor: a study of cytologic features of six cases diagnosed by fine-needle aspiration. *Diagn Cytopathol.* 2001;25:172–176.
2. Ali SZ, Hoon V, Hoda S, Heelan R, Zakowski MF. Solitary fibrous tumor. A cytologic-histologic study with clinical, radiologic, and immunohistochemical correlations. *Cancer.* 1997;81(2): 116–121.

CASE

106

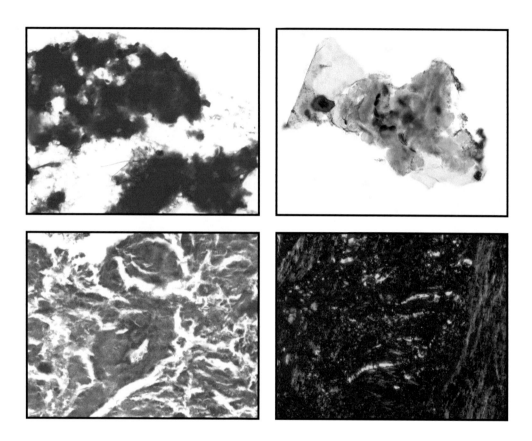

Clinical History

A 77-year-old woman with a long smoking history presents with shortness of breath. Chest x-rays show multiple nodular densities in both lungs. Ultrasound-guided transthoracic lung fine needle aspiration.

Choose the Best Diagnosis

a. Chondroid metaplasia

b. Amyloid nodule

c. Necrotic non-small cell carcinoma

d. Normal lung tissue

e. Pulmonary abscess

ANSWER AND BRIEF DISCUSSION

b. Amyloid Nodule

Globules of amorphous waxy material are seen throughout the smears. The smears are largely acellular. Apple green birefringence was seen on Congo red staining.

The clinical presentation is worrisome for a number of different entities including lung carcinoma, metastatic disease to the lung, and perhaps infection. However, the sampled material is not diagnostic for any of these. The amorphous globules are amyloid, as confirmed by Congo red staining. Amyloidosis in a nodular bronchial or nodular parenchymal distribution can appear as solitary or multiple radiographic lesions. Amyloidosis also can present diffusely in a vascular distribution or in a diffuse alveolar septal pattern.

Reference

1. Dundore PA, Aisner SC, Templeton PA, Krasna MJ, White CS, Seidman JD. Nodular pulmonary amyloidosis: diagnosis by fine-needle aspiration cytology and a review of the literature. *Diagn Cytopathol*. 1993;9:562–564.

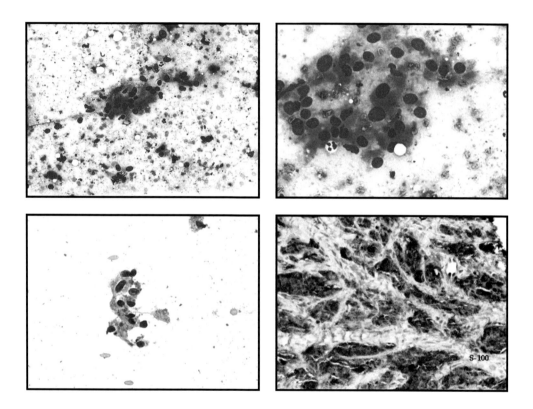

Clinical History

Fine needle aspiration of a 3-cm forearm lesion in a 4-year-old girl. An S-100 protein immunostain is provided.

Choose the Best Diagnosis

a. Langerhans cell histiocytosis

b. Granular cell tumor (GCT)

c. Alveolar soft part sarcoma

d. Epithelioid sarcoma

e. Merkel cell carcinoma

ANSWER AND BRIEF DISCUSSION

b. Granular Cell Tumor (GCT)

The aspirate shows scattered round to polygonal cells with round eccentric nuclei, conspicuous nucleoli, and abundant granular cytoplasm. Many naked nuclei are noted, and granular debris is present in the background. The cells were immunoreactive for S-100 protein.

The cytomorphologic and immunohistochemical findings described above are consistent with GCT. The origin of GCTs is still being debated, but most writers on the subject favor a Schwann cell origin. GCTs typically occur in adults, but can be seen in children. The most common site of occurrence is the tongue, but these tumors have a wide range of distribution including the extremities. Nearly all cases are positive for S-100 protein. Cases associated with epithelial surfaces sometimes have secondary epithelial hyperplastic changes that may be incorrectly diagnosed as carcinoma. Although the vast majority of GCTs have a benign clinical course, distant metastases have been reported.

Reference

1. Liu K, Madden JF, Olatidoye BA, Dodd LG. Features of benign granular cell tumor on fine needle aspiration. *Acta Cytol.* 1999;43:552–557.

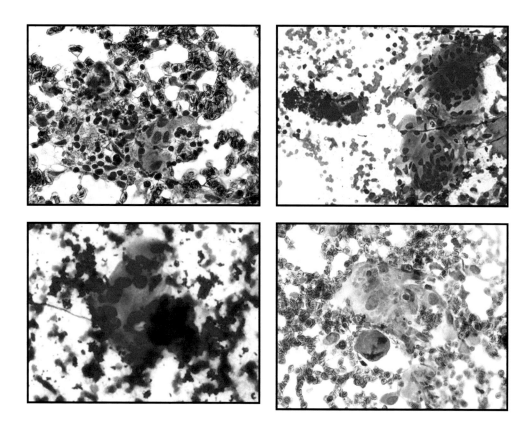

Clinical History

A 59-year-old woman has diffuse myalgias, fevers, chills, and rigors in the evenings associated with left neck and left ear pain. Ultrasound of the thyroid shows a large heterogeneous right lobe. It is not clear to the radiologist whether this represented a large nodule replacing the entire right lobe or an enlarged right lobe due to a diffuse process. Ultrasound-guided fine needle aspiration.

Choose the Best Diagnosis

    a. Adenomatoid nodule

    b. Hashimoto thyroiditis

    c. Metastatic breast ductal carcinoma

    d. Suspicious for a follicular neoplasm

    e. Granulomatous thyroiditis

ANSWER AND BRIEF DISCUSSION

e. Granulomatous Thyroiditis

In the background, there is colloid mixed with scattered follicular epithelium. Numerous histiocytes and occasional giant cells also are identified. Rare giant cells appear to be engulfing clumps of colloid.

There is no neoplastic cell population present. The presence of giant cells and histiocytes is consistent with granulomatous thyroiditis. Microbial cultures are recommended to rule out acid-fast bacteria and fungal organisms. Other entities under the umbrella of granulomatous thyroiditis include palpation thyroiditis and sarcoidosis. Despite the lack of a lymphocytic background, one final possibility is deQuervain thyroiditis, given the classic clinical picture of a middle-aged woman with recent history of fever and subsequent neck pain with dysphagia.

References

1. Baloch ZW, LiVolsi VA, Asa SL, et al. Diagnostic terminology and morphologic criteria for cytologic diagnosis of thyroid lesions: a synopsis of the National Cancer Institute thyroid fine-needle aspiration state of the science conference. *Diagn Cytopathol.* 2008;36:425–437.
2. Cibas ES, Ali SZ. The Bethesda system for reporting thyroid cytopathology. *Thyroid.* 2009;19: 1159–1165.

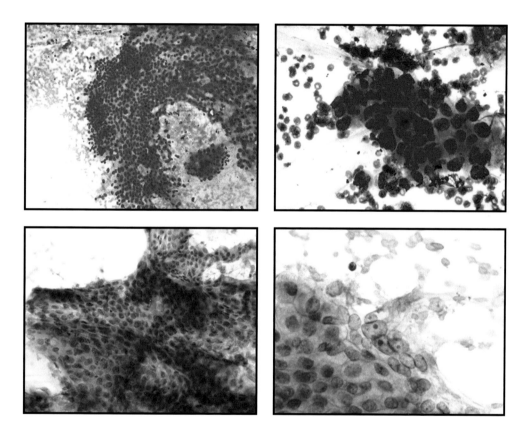

Clinical History

A 49-year-old man with obstructive jaundice found to have a 5-cm mass of the head of the pancreas. Transabdominal ultrasound-guided fine needle aspiration (FNA) of the pancreas.

Choose the Best Diagnosis

a. Pancreatitis

b. Pancreatic pseudocyst

c. Pancreatic adenocarcinoma

d. Intraductal papillary mucinous neoplasm

e. Pancreatic neuroendocrine tumor

ANSWER AND BRIEF DISCUSSION

c. Pancreatic Adenocarcinoma

The aspirate is cellular and consists of sheets of predominantly ductal-type cells. The sheets have architectural disorder, with uneven spacing of nuclei and crowding. At higher power, many of the ductal cells have prominent nucleoli and nuclear membrane irregularities.

The first clue to the diagnosis in this case is that the lesion is cellular and dominated by sheets of ductal cells. Architectural disorder within the sheets is another feature seen in carcinoma. High-power clues are the irregular nuclear contours and macronucleoli. Pancreatic adenocarcinoma must be distinguished from pancreatitis. These two diseases have significant clinical overlap, and both can present with obstructive jaundice, pain, and weight loss. FNAs of pancreatitis are sparsely cellular and typically show a ductal predominance. Significant nuclear atypia can be seen in pancreatitis, but markedly irregular nuclear contours and macronucleoli are indicative of carcinoma.

Reference

1. Bellizzi AM, Stelow EB. Pancreatic cytopathology: a practical approach and review. *Arch Pathol Lab Med.* 2009;133:388–404.

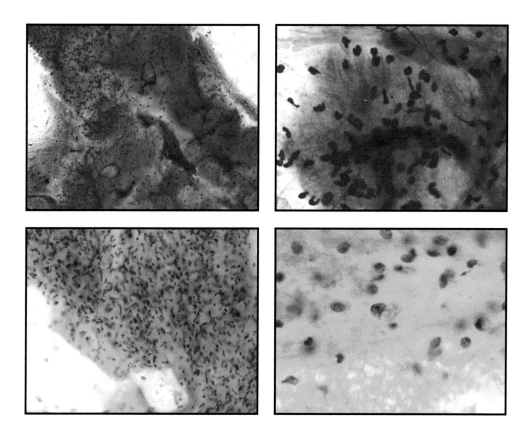

Clinical History

A previously healthy 41-year-old man presents with a 10-cm soft tissue leg mass that does not involve the femur. Fine needle aspiration of the lesion.

Choose the Best Diagnosis

a. Nodular fasciitis (NF)

b. Ischemic fasciitis

c. Myxoid liposarcoma (ML)

d. Myxoid chondrosarcoma

e. Myositis ossificans

ANSWER AND BRIEF DISCUSSION

c. Myxoid Liposarcoma (ML)

The aspirates show abundant myxoid material with scattered spindle cells and occasional lipoblasts. The lipoblasts have nuclear indentions due to cytoplasmic vacuoles. The spindled cells and lipoblasts are clustered around complex branching capillary networks.

This case illustrates the characteristic features of ML. ML is the most common type of liposarcoma and shows a marked predilection for the lower extremities, particularly the thigh. Even without the lipoblasts, the rich branching capillary network is very characteristic of ML. NF and ischemic fasciitis are both benign mesenchymal proliferative processes that can be misinterpreted as sarcomatous. NF is characterized clinically by rapid growth (days to weeks) and is sometimes associated with local trauma. Ischemic fasciitis typically occurs in immobilized patients in the sacrum and is characterized by zones of necrosis surrounded by neovessels and proliferating myofibroblasts. For either condition to cause a 10-cm mass lesion would be unusual.

References

1. Gonzalez-Campora R, Otal-Salaverri C, Hevia-Vazquez A, Munoz-Munoz G, Garrido-Cintado A, Galera-Davidson H. Fine needle aspiration in myxoid tumors of the soft tissues. *Acta Cytol.* 1990;34:179–191.
2. Wakely PE, Jr., Geisinger KR, Cappellari JO, Silverman JF, Frable WJ. Fine-needle aspiration cytopathology of soft tissue: chondromyxoid and myxoid lesions. *Diagn Cytopathol.* 1995;12: 101–105.

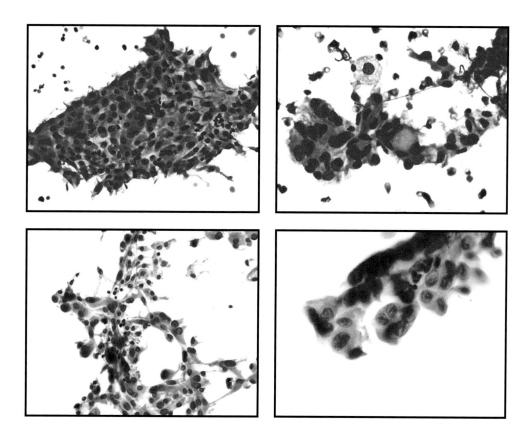

Clinical History

Thyroid fine needle aspiration in a 28-year-old woman.

Choose the Best Diagnosis

    a. Benign, consistent with an adenomatoid nodule

    b. Suspicious for a follicular neoplasm

    c. Suspicious for malignancy

    d. Anaplastic thyroid carcinoma

    e. Medullary thyroid carcinoma

ANSWER AND BRIEF DISCUSSION

c. Suspicious for Malignancy

The aspirates are cellular and show numerous monolayered tissue fragments with essentially no background colloid. The epithelial tissue fragments have moderate atypia and architectural disorder. The nuclei are crowded and enlarged with some discernible nucleoli. Occasional grooves are present, as well as microfollicular formations. Admixed among the epithelial cells are numerous small lymphocytes and scattered histiocytes. Intranuclear inclusions and psammoma bodies are not identified.

This is a really challenging case. Though the cellularity and disordered architecture are concerning for papillary thyroid carcinoma (PTC), the nuclear features do not fulfill diagnostic criteria. Interpreting cytologic aspirates of proliferative epithelial lesions in a background of chronic lymphocytic thyroiditis is a common diagnostic dilemma in thyroid cytology. For a cytologic diagnosis of PTC in the background of Hashimoto thyroiditis, the presence of minimal criteria is mandatory. After much debate, we equivocated in this case. Subsequent excision was signed out as atypical papillary hyperplasia in a background of Hashimoto thyroiditis.

References

1. Baloch ZW, Cibas ES, Clark DP, et al. The National Cancer Institute thyroid fine needle aspiration state of the science conference: a summation. *Cytojournal.* 2008;5:6.
2. Cibas ES, Ali SZ. The Bethesda system for reporting thyroid cytopathology. *Thyroid.* 2009;19: 1159–1165.

CASE

112

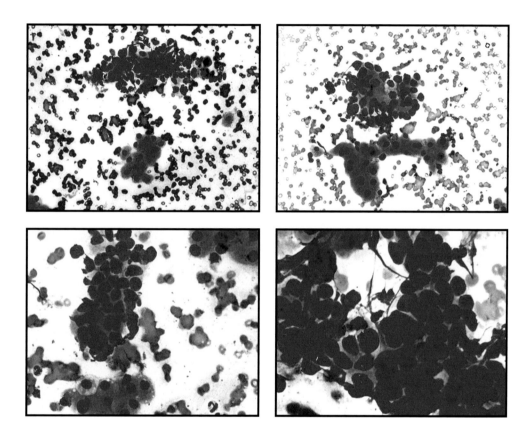

Liver fine needle aspiration in a 62-year-old woman.

Choose the Best Diagnosis

a. Poorly differentiated hepatocellular carcinoma (HCC)

b. Adenocarcinoma, favor cholangiocarcinoma

c. Ductular proliferation consistent with obstruction

d. Atypical fragments strongly suspicious for carcinoma

e. Reactive changes consistent with viral hepatitis

ANSWER AND BRIEF DISCUSSION

b. Adenocarcinoma, Favor Cholangiocarcinoma

The aspirate shows fragments and single benign hepatocytes with adjacent cohesive groups of overtly malignant epithelial cells. The malignant cells are architecturally disordered with nuclear crowding and overlap. The cells have enlarged pleomorphic nuclei and scant cytoplasm. The background is relatively clean.

The cytomorphologic features described are beyond the realm of reactive and are diagnostic of adenocarcinoma. The patient had a history of cholangiocarcinoma, and this was a recurrent lesion. While HCC should be considered, the malignant cells bare no similarity to hepatocytes, and no vascular architecture/endothelial wrapping was present. Metastatic adenocarcinoma would also be a consideration depending on the clinical context and in most cases cannot be differentiated from cholangiocarcinoma by cytomorphologic features alone.

Reference

1. Bottles K, Cohen MB. An approach to fine-needle aspiration biopsy diagnosis of hepatic masses. *Diagn Cytopathol.* 1991;7:204–210.

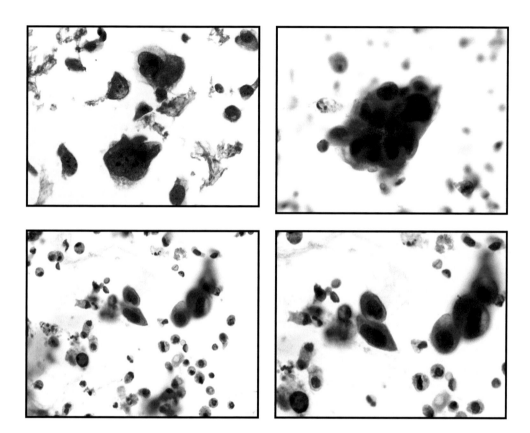

Clinical History

Ileal conduit (neobladder) contents in a 73-year-old man who is status post radical cystectomy for urothelial carcinoma.

Choose the Best Diagnosis

a. Polyoma virus cytopathic effect

b. Degenerative atypia, no malignancy identified

c. Benign ileal conduit contents

d. High-grade urothelial carcinoma

e. Renal cell carcinoma

ANSWER AND BRIEF DISCUSSION

d. High-Grade Urothelial Carcinoma

The specimen shows fragments and single malignant cells with background degenerated enterocytes and debris. The malignant cells are moderately sized and contain deeply staining hyperchromatic nuclei with irregular nuclear contours. The cells have a moderate amount of cytoplasm that appears focally vacuolated.

The cytologic features described above are consistent with urothelial carcinoma. Urothelial carcinoma accounts for 90% of primary tumors of the bladder and has been linked with smoking and environmental exposure to aniline dyes. The most important prognostic indicator is surgical stage, and the 5-year survival rate for deeply invasive urothelial carcinoma is between 45% and 55%.

References

1. Rosenthal DL, VandenBussche CJ, Burroughs FH, Sathiyamoorthy S, Guan H, Owens C. The Johns Hopkins Hospital template for urologic cytology samples: part i-creating the template. *Cancer Cytopathol*. 2013;121(1):15–20.
2. Owens CL, VandenBussche CJ, Burroughs FH, Rosenthal DL. A review of reporting systems and terminology for urine cytology. *Cancer Cytopathol*. 2013;121(1):9–14.

CASE

114

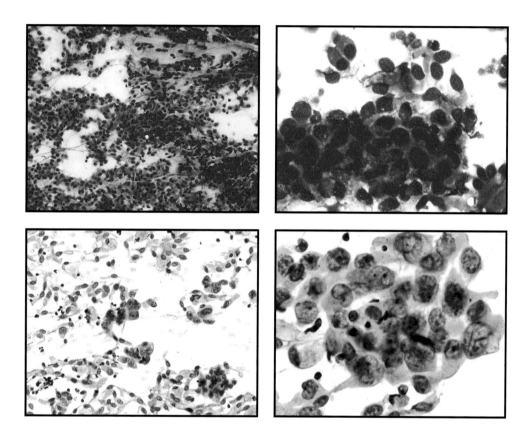

Clinical History

Bronchoscopic wash in a 46-year-old man with a 2.5-cm lung mass. The patient has a 20-pack-year smoking history and an unintentional 15-pound weight loss over the last 3 months. Transbronchial tissue biopsy directed at the mass is negative for malignancy.

Choose the Best Diagnosis

a. Reserve cell hyperplasia

b. Ciliated bronchial epithelial cells with reactive changes

c. Non-small cell carcinoma

d. Atypical squamous metaplasia

e. Small cell carcinoma

ANSWER AND BRIEF DISCUSSION

c. Non-Small Cell Carcinoma

The specimen shows predominantly polarized, benign respiratory epithelial cells with terminal bars and cilia. However, there is a second population of epithelial cells admixed among the benign cells that have larger, pleomorphic nuclei and architectural abnormalities including crowding and overlap. Higher power reveals that the atypical cells have irregular nuclear contours and clumped chromatin. Some of the atypical cells have finely vacuolated cytoplasm, suggesting glandular differentiation.

This is a challenging case, but the smaller population of atypical cells fulfills criteria for malignancy. At the time of the lung fine needle aspiration, this patient had radiographic evidence of metastatic disease with lesions in his liver and one of his adrenal glands. There was an apparent sampling error with the biopsy that was negative for malignancy. The patient was started on chemotherapy with initial tumor response radiographically (including the lung lesion). However, the patient ultimately died of metastatic disease 9 months after diagnosis.

Reference

1. Solomon DA, Solliday NH, Gracey DR. Cytology in fiberoptic bronchoscopy: comparison of bronchial brushing, washing and post-bronchoscopy sputum. *Chest.* 1974;65(6):616–619.

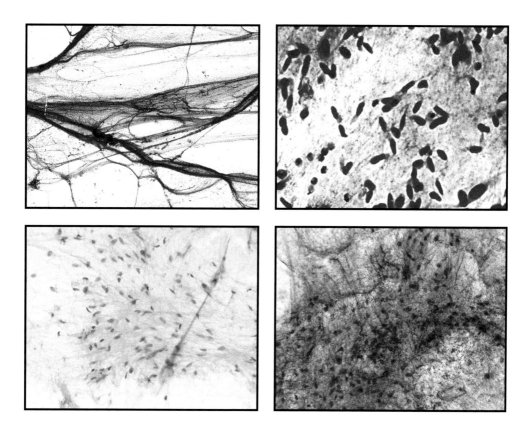

Clinical History

A 34-year-old woman with a 6-cm mass on the anterior aspect of her right lower leg. Fine needle aspiration (FNA). An S-100 protein immunohistochemical stain was negative (not pictured).

Choose the Best Diagnosis

a. Myxoid liposarcoma

b. Myxoid chondrosarcoma

c. Myxoma

d. Myxofibrosarcoma

e. Malignant melanoma

ANSWER AND BRIEF DISCUSSION

c. Myxoma

Numerous spindle cells are found in a myxoid background. Although most of the cells are bland, some have mild cytologic atypia with nuclear pleomorphism and nuclear enlargement. No blood vessels or mitotic figures are seen.

The smears and cell block lack vascularity that might suggest myxoid liposarcoma; myxoid liposarcoma is characterized by prominent vascularity that is seen on histologic sections as a "chicken wire" pattern. The absence of chondroblasts are unfavorable for myxoid chondrosarcoma. While this FNA may represent a benign process (ie, myxoma), the findings of focal atypia are concerning enough for a low-grade sarcoma that we equivocated with our diagnosis. Subsequent biopsies of the mass resulted in the diagnosis of a myxoma. Although the lesion has areas of cellularity with focal nuclear enlargement, overall, it does not have sufficient vascularity or atypia to warrant the diagnosis of a sarcoma.

References

1. Wakely PE Jr Geisinger KR, Cappellari JO, Silverman JF, Frable WJ. Fine-needle aspiration cytopathology of soft tissue: chondromyxoid and myxoid lesions. *Diagn Cytopathol.* 1995;12:101–105.
2. Wakely PE Jr. Myxomatous soft tissue tumors: correlation of cytopathology and histopathology. *Ann Diagn Pathol.* 1999;3:227–242.

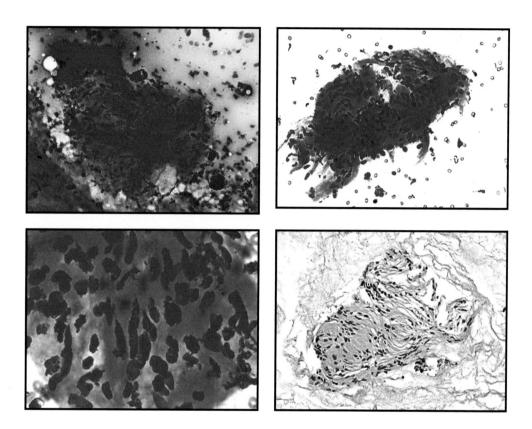

Clinical History

A 70-year-old man presents with a 1-year history of a growing mass on the right side of his face. Physical exam reveals a mobile, 3-cm retromandibular parotid mass, and neurologic exam shows no voluntary right eye closure. Fine needle aspiration of right parotid mass.

Choose the Best Diagnosis

a. Adenoid cystic carcinoma

b. Pleomorphic adenoma

c. Leiomyosarcoma

d. Schwannoma

e. Spindle cell neoplasm, consistent with metastatic malignant melanoma

ANSWER AND BRIEF DISCUSSION

d. Schwannoma

The aspirate shows numerous spindle cells with club-shaped nuclei that cling together and do not appear to smear out as single cells. No mitotic activity is seen. Immunohistochemical staining showed that the cells were reactive for S-100 protein (not shown).

While the clinical history of a salivary gland mass with facial nerve paralysis might suggest adenoid cystic carcinoma, the aspirate demonstrates no characteristic basaloid cells or hyaline globules. The cell block and immunostain are very helpful; S-100 protein-positive Verocay bodies lead us to the diagnosis of schwannoma. In the proper clinical setting (ie, previous history), one might entertain the diagnosis of metastatic spindle cell melanoma, but the cells in this aspirate are very bland and have no mitotic activity. Subsequent surgical resection confirmed the diagnosis of schwannoma.

References

1. Yu GH, Sack MJ, Baloch Z, Gupta PK. Difficulties in the fine needle aspiration (FNA) diagnosis of schwannoma. *Cytopathology.* 1999;10:186–194.
2. Assad L, Treaba D, Ariga R, et al. Fine-needle aspiration of parotid gland schwannomas mimicking pleomorphic adenoma: a report of two cases. *Diagn Cytopathol.* 2004;30:39–40.
3. Kapila K, Mathur S, Verma K. Schwannomas: a pitfall in the diagnosis of pleomorphic adenomas on fine-needle aspiration cytology. *Diagn Cytopathol.* 2002;27:53–59.

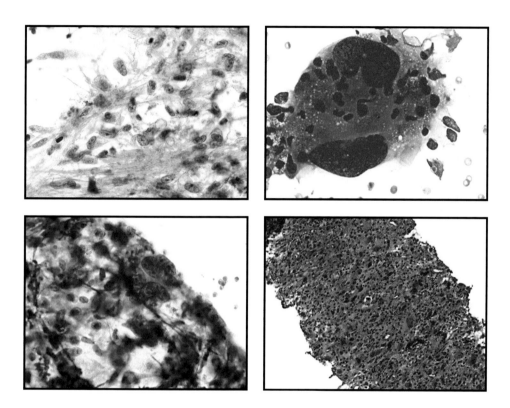

Clinical History

A 53-year-old man presents with an enlarging 6-cm liver mass identified on abdominal CT scan. He has a history of chordoma of the sacrum initially resected 18 months prior to presentation; approximately 1 year after that procedure, the tumor recurred in the sacrum and showed extensive areas of dedifferentiated high-grade sarcoma. Fine needle aspiration of liver mass with core biopsy.

Choose the Best Diagnosis

a. Metastatic high-grade pleomorphic sarcoma

b. Hepatocellular carcinoma (HCC)

c. Metastatic melanoma

d. Metastatic adenocarcinoma consistent with colonic primary

e. Hemangioma

ANSWER AND BRIEF DISCUSSION

a. Metastatic High-Grade Pleomorphic Sarcoma

Numerous large, pleomorphic cells with wildly atypical mitoses and highly atypical nuclei are seen in the smear and in the core biopsy. The nuclei are many, many times the size of lymphocytes, and chromatin is very coarse with multiple nucleoli. High-grade features are clearly evident.

The cells identified in the liver aspirate are morphologically similar to those seen in the prior dedifferentiated sarcoma. In the absence of this history, the differential for pleomorphic pink cell neoplasms in the liver includes melanoma, HCC, and adrenal cortical carcinoma.

Reference

1. Willen H, Akerman M, Carlen B. Fine needle aspiration (FNA) in the diagnosis of soft tissue tumours; a review of 22 years experience. *Cytopathology*. 1995;6:236–247.

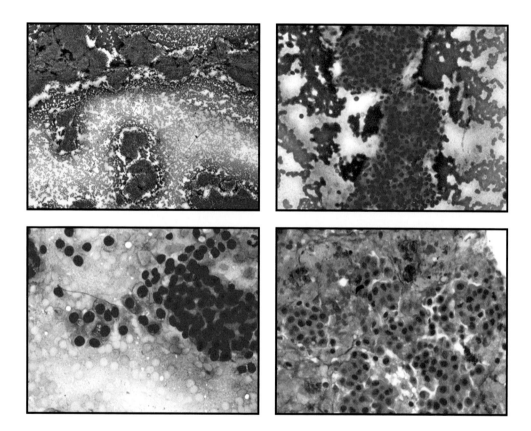

Clinical History

Transabdominal ultrasound-guided fine needle aspiration of a 3-cm pancreatic mass in a 57-year-old woman.

Choose the Best Diagnosis

    a. Acinar cell carcinoma

    b. Ductal adenocarcinoma

    c. Pancreatic neuroendocrine tumor (PanNET)

    d. Chronic pancreatitis

    e. Solid pseudopapillary neoplasm

ANSWER AND BRIEF DISCUSSION

a. Acinar Cell Carcinoma

The aspirate is cellular and shows cohesive fragments of a monomorphic population of cells. The fragments are crowded and disordered, and the cells have round nuclei that are often eccentrically placed, increased N/C ratios, and granular cytoplasm. No ductal elements are appreciated.

The fact that only one cell type is present indicates that this is a neoplastic process. The main differential in this case is between PanNET and acinar cell carcinoma. Without immunohistochemical stains, that distinction would be extremely difficult on cytomorphologic grounds alone. Acinar cell carcinomas of the pancreas account for less than 5% of pancreatic malignancies and have a slight male predominance. The tumors can have acinar or solid growth patterns and tend to have round to oval nuclei that are relatively uniform. Immunohistochemical stains for trypsin, chymotrypsin, amylase, and lipase are frequently positive. The clinical syndrome of disseminated fat necrosis, polyarthralgia, and eosinophilia has been associated with these tumors and is a consequence of the secretion of lipase or other digestive enzymes. The prognosis is poor, with most patients dying within a few months of diagnosis.

Reference

1. Stelow EB, Bardales RH, Shami VM, et al. Cytology of pancreatic acinar cell carcinoma. *Diagn Cytopathol*. 2006;34:367–372.

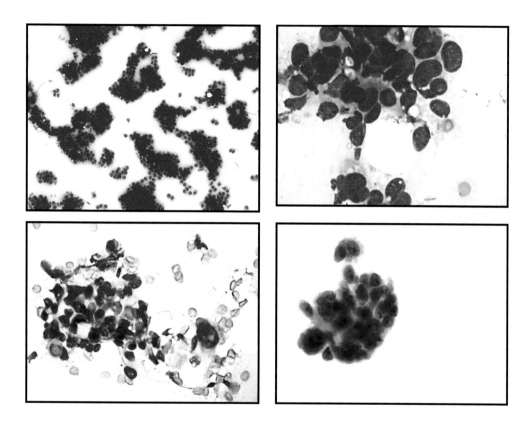

Clinical History

A 32-year-old woman presents with a new breast mass found on mammography. Ultrasound demonstrates an 8-mm hypoechoic nodule. Ultrasound-guided fine needle aspiration of the breast.

Choose the Best Diagnosis

a. Mammary carcinoma

b. Fibroadenoma

c. Fibrocystic changes

d. Intraductal papilloma

e. Lactational changes

ANSWER AND BRIEF DISCUSSION

a. Mammary Carcinoma

Although the smear is not overly hypercellular, there are many fragments of large, hyperchromatic cells in a background of fat and occasional blood. The cells are pleomorphic, with prominent nucleoli and coarse chromatin. The nuclei are up to 4 to 5 times larger than neighboring red blood cells.

A diagnosis of carcinoma is supported by the classic malignant features; subclassification is difficult in this sample, although a ductal carcinoma is favored due to hints of gland-forming behavior. Subsequent core biopsy showed infiltrating moderately differentiated ductal carcinoma.

Reference

1. Stanley MW, Sidawy MK, Sanchez MA, Stahl RE, Goldfischer M. Current issues in breast cytopathology. *Am J Clin Pathol.* 2000;113:S49–S75.

CASE

120

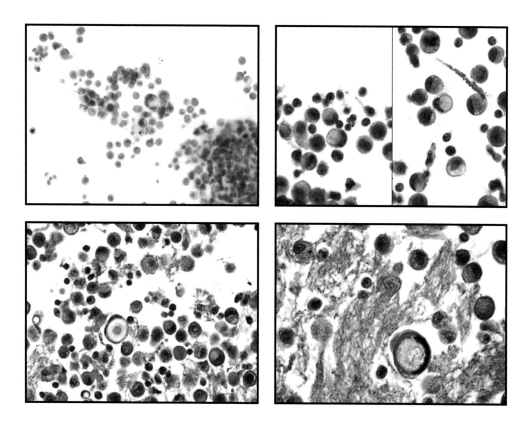

Clinical History

A 66-year-old man presents with a 6-month history of progressively worsening dysphagia with liquids and solid foods, a 12-pound (5.4 kg) weight loss, and abdominal distension. Abdominal paracentesis (cytospin).

Choose the Best Diagnosis

a. Reactive mesothelial cells and chronic inflammatory cells

b. Mesothelioma

c. Carcinoma with signet ring cell features

d. Peritoneal mucinous carcinomatosis

e. Granulomatous inflammation

ANSWER AND BRIEF DISCUSSION

c. Carcinoma With Signet Ring Cell Features

Numerous large discohesive single cells are seen in the fluid. These cells have enlarged nuclei that are pushed to one side by a cytoplasmic vacuole in a "signet ring" configuration. Immunohistochemical studies showed that the cells are immunoreactive for CK7, CK20, CD15 (LeuM1), and BerEp4. The cells are nonreactive for calretinin. Mucicarmine stain is positive.

Subsequent biopsy of an esophageal stricture showed a signet ring cell carcinoma at the gastroesophageal junction, with cells very similar to those seen in the effusion. The distinction between metastatic adenocarcinoma and mesothelial cells (reactive or malignant) in an effusion often is facilitated by immunohistochemical studies. Mesothelial cells are immunoreactive for calretinin and nonreactive for CD15 (LeuM1) and BerEp4, while the reverse is true for adenocarcinomas. Other helpful immunohistochemical stains include CEA and B72.3. Both tend to be immunoreactive in adenocarcinomas and nonreactive in mesothelial cells.

Reference

1. Fetsch PA, Abati A. Immunocytochemistry in effusion cytology: a contemporary review. *Cancer.* 2001;93:293–308.

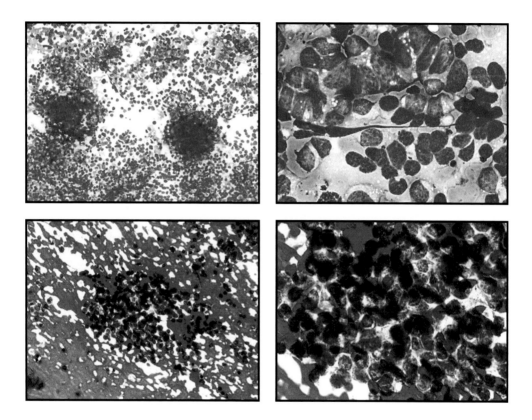

Clinical History

An 8-year-old boy with a history of Wilms' tumor presents with ascites and multiple hypodense lesions in the liver on abdominal CT. Fine needle aspiration of liver mass.

Choose the Best Diagnosis

    a. Hepatocellular carcinoma

    b. Metastatic Wilms' tumor

    c. Angiosarcoma

    d. Normal hepatic tissue

    e. Non-Hodgkin lymphoma

ANSWER AND BRIEF DISCUSSION

b. Metastatic Wilms' Tumor

The aspirate is hypercellular and comprises many atypical cells with high N/C ratio, fine to slightly coarse chromatin, and nuclear molding. No obvious tubules or stromal cells are identified.

Wilms' tumor is often easily diagnosed in the presence of all three components (epithelium, stroma, and blastema). The cells seen here represent a poorly differentiated malignant neoplasm that, given the history, is most consistent with metastatic Wilms' tumor, blastema component. Immunohistochemical stains for WT-1 and thyroid transcription factor-1 were noncontributory due to lack of tissue on the core biopsy.

References

1. Radhika S, Bakshi A, Rajwanshi A, et al. Cytopathology of uncommon malignant renal neoplasms in the pediatric age group. *Diagn Cytopathol.* 2005;32:281–286.
2. Portugal R, Barroca H. Clear cell sarcoma, cellular mesoblastic nephroma and metanephric adenoma: cytological features and differential diagnosis with Wilms tumour. *Cytopathology.* 2008;19:80–85.

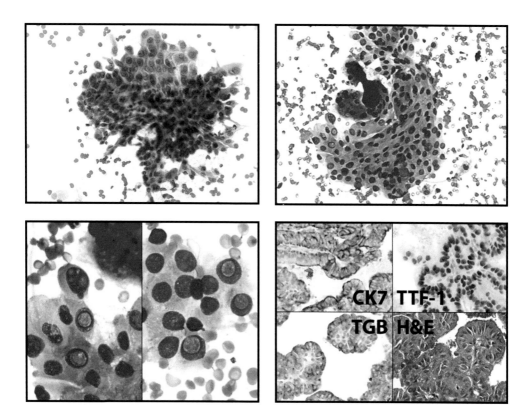

Clinical History

A 49-year-old man presents with a 5-week history of pain in the medial left thigh that is worse with weight-bearing and stair-climbing. Past medical history is significant for a thyroid nodule removed 6 years ago that, per patient report, was benign. Fine needle aspiration of a lytic left femoral lesion.

Choose the Best Diagnosis

a. Plasma cell myeloma

b. Metastatic adenocarcinoma consistent with prostatic primary

c. Metastatic adenocarcinoma of lung

d. Metastatic papillary thyroid carcinoma (PTC)

e. Osteomyelitis

ANSWER AND BRIEF DISCUSSION

d. Metastatic Papillary Thyroid Carcinoma (PTC)

Papanicolaou and Diff-Quik stains show tissue fragments with cells having enlarged round to oval nuclei and prominent nuclear pseudoinclusions. Hematoxylin and eosin-stained cell block material shows papillary architecture. Immunohistochemical stains show that the tumor cells are reactive for CK7, thyroid transcription factor-1 (TTF-1), thyroglobulin, and DPC-4 (not shown). Additional immunohistochemical stains (not shown) revealed that the cells are nonreactive for CK20, RCC, PSA, and PSAP.

A lytic lesion in the bone of an older patient is metastasis until proven otherwise. Potential primary sites in the differential diagnosis are rendered less likely, given the nonreactive PSA and PSAP (prostate) and RCC (kidney), while a DPC-4 stain is informative for pancreatic adenocarcinoma only when it is nonreactive. TTF-1 (nuclear) and CK7 (membrane) immunoreactivity suggest lung and thyroid, while thyroglobulin positivity (cytoplasmic) makes the diagnosis of metastatic PTC. A subsequent total thyroidectomy revealed PTC. The previously resected thyroid tissue from 6 years ago was not available for review.

Reference

1. Dinneen SF, Valimaki MJ, Bergstalh EJ, Goellner JR, Gorman CA, Hay ID. Distant metastases in papillary thyroid carcinoma: 100 cases observed at one institution during 5 decades. *J Clin Endocrinol Metab.* 1995;80:2041–2045.

CASE

123

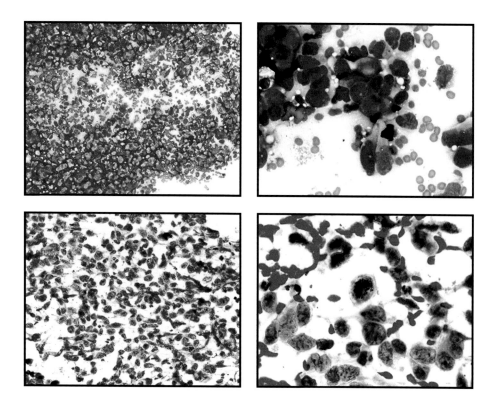

Clinical History

A 71-year-old man with a history of hormone-refractory prostate cancer presents with a pelvic mass. Fine needle aspiration of pelvic lesion. Immunohistochemical stains performed on the cell block show that the cells are reactive for CK AE1/3 (pancytokeratin) and CD56, but are nonreactive for PSA, PSAP, CD45, and thyroid transcription factor-1. The patient has never been a smoker.

Choose the Best Diagnosis

a. High-grade lymphoma

b. High-grade sarcoma

c. Metastatic carcinoma with small cell features, favor prostate origin

d. Metastatic carcinoma with small cell features, favor lung origin

e. Metastatic melanoma

ANSWER AND BRIEF DISCUSSION

c. Metastatic Carcinoma With Small Cell Features, Favor Prostate Origin

The aspirates show a monomorphic population of malignant cells. The cells are hyperchromatic and have increased N/C ratios with scant cytoplasm. The chromatin pattern is finely granular, and some of the cells show nuclear molding. Abundant mitotic figures are identified.

The findings are diagnostic of malignancy, and there are morphologic features and immunohistochemical evidence of small cell neuroendocrine differentiation. Small cell carcinoma of the prostate may arise de novo or in association with a more typical adenocarcinoma. It is not uncommon to see small cell phenotype in metastases of high-grade prostate adenocarcinomas. Small cell carcinoma of any organ has significant morphologic overlap with high-grade lymphomas, and as such, excluding hematopoietic origin is prudent. In our case, CD45 was negative and AE1/3 was reactive. Despite the lack of reactivity with prostate-specific antigens, the most likely site of origin in this case is the prostate. Not infrequently, metastatic high-grade carcinoma of prostatic origin will fail to label with PSA and PSAP. In such cases, serum PSA may be helpful. Also, small cell carcinoma of the lung occurs almost exclusively in smokers.

References

1. Caraway NP, Fanning CV, Shin HJ, Amato RJ. Metastatic small-cell carcinoma of the prostate diagnosed by fine-needle aspiration biopsy. *Diagn Cytopathol*. 1998;19:12–16.
2. Wang W, Epstein JI. Small cell carcinoma of the prostate. A morphologic and immunohistochemical study of 95 cases. *Am J Surg Pathol*. 2008;32:65–71.
3. Parwani AV, Ali SZ. Prostatic adenocarcinoma metastases mimicking small cell carcinoma on fine-needle aspiration. *Diagn Cytopathol*. 2002;27(2):75–79.

CASE

124

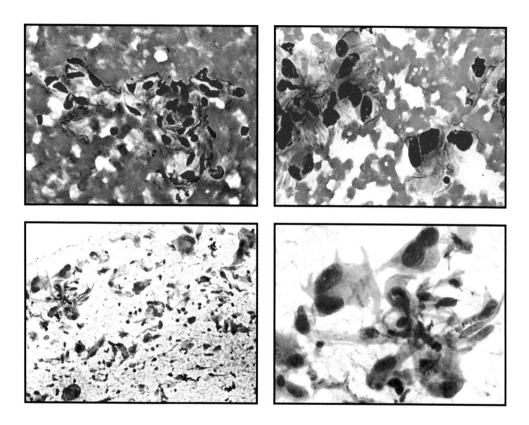

Clinical History

A 72-year-old white male presents with a 1 to 2 month history of left back pain. The patient had a well-differentiated liposarcoma resected 7 years ago. Abdominal CT revealed several large fatty masses in the retroperitoneum. Fine needle aspiration of retroperitoneal mass.

Choose the Best Diagnosis

a. Granulomatous inflammation

b. Nodular fasciitis

c. Solitary fibrous tumor

d. Sarcoma consistent with recurrence of liposarcoma

e. Desmoid fibromatosis

ANSWER AND BRIEF DISCUSSION

d. Sarcoma Consistent With Recurrence of Liposarcoma

Scattered tissue fragments and single cells are seen in a background of numerous red blood cells. Bland spindle cells are admixed with large, pleomorphic, bizarre-shaped binucleated cells with coarse chromatin and occasional prominent nucleoli.

The degree of atypia and pleomorphism are compatible with a high-grade process. Although no lipoblasts are definitively identified, the history and location make recurrent liposarcoma the most likely diagnosis. The presence of significant pleomorphism suggests dedifferentiation (dedifferentiated liposarcoma).

References

1. Willen H, Akerman M, Carlen B. Fine needle aspiration (FNA) in the diagnosis of soft tissue tumours; a review of 22 years experience. *Cytopathology*. 1995;6:236–247.
2. Walaas L, Kindblom LG. Lipomatous tumors: a correlative cytologic and histologic study of 27 tumors examined by fine needle aspiration cytology. *Human Pathol*. 1985;16:6–18.

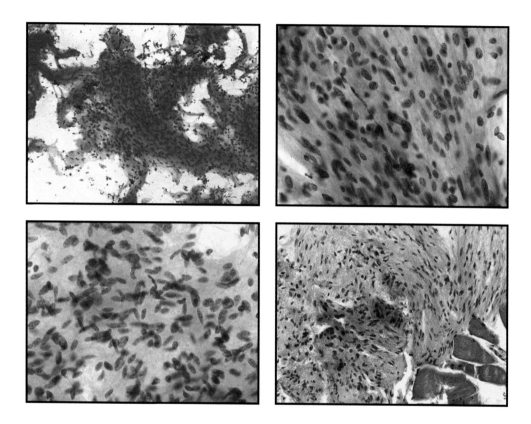

Clinical History

Fine needle aspiration of a 4.2-cm well-defined lesion within the peroneus longus muscle in a 59-year-old woman.

Choose the Best Diagnosis

a. Lipoma

b. Intramuscular myxoma

c. Schwannoma

d. Fibromatosis

e. Synovial sarcoma

ANSWER AND BRIEF DISCUSSION

c. Schwannoma

At low power, the lesion consists of a cohesive fragment of bland spindle cells. Upon closer examination, some nuclei are oval shaped, while others appear more wavy and serpentine. Nuclear pleomorphism is minimal, and the chromatin pattern is finely dispersed. The cytoplasm appears indistinct in these smears. Importantly, the nuclei are embedded in a distinctly fibrillary matrix, and in this case, no myxoid matrix is identified. While cell block preparation artifact partially disrupts the architecture, areas of palisading can be identified, and some regions appear more cellular than others (Antoni A/Antoni B).

Reactivity for S-100 protein on immunoperoxidase staining is confirmatory for a nerve sheath tumor; the bland nuclear features exclude a malignant peripheral nerve sheath tumor. In some instances, the matrix may appear myxoid, leading to myxoid soft tissue lesions entering the differential diagnosis. Long-standing schwannomas can undergo "ancient" change, which can result in severe nuclear atypia, mimicking a malignant process such as sarcoma or carcinoma. The absence of adipocytes excludes lipoma. Extra-abdominal fibromatosis (desmoid tumor) should be considered as a possibility in certain anatomic locations. In fibromatosis, the nuclei are fusiform, and cells are positive for actin, negative for S-100 protein, and demonstrate positive nuclear beta-catenin immunoperoxidase staining.

References

1. Domanski HA. Fine-needle aspiration challenges of soft tissue lesions: diagnostic challenges. *Diagn Cytopathol.* 2007;35(12):768–773.
2. Owens CL, Sharma R, Ali SZ. Deep fibromatosis (desmoid tumor). *Cancer.* 2007;111(3):166–172.

INDEX BY CASE DIAGNOSIS

INDEX BY CASE TOPIC

Printed in the United States
By Bookmasters